D0386392

EPILEPSY
and the Family

A NEW GUIDE

EPILEPSY

and the Family

A NEW GUIDE

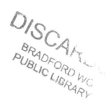

Richard Lechtenberg, M.D.

HARVARD UNIVERSITY PRESS
Cambridge, Massachusetts
London, England
1999

Library of Congress Cataloging-in-Publication Data

Lechtenberg, Richard.
  Epilepsy and the family : a new guide / Richard Lechtenberg.
    p. cm.
  Includes bibliographical references and index.
  ISBN 0-674-25897-5
  1. Epileptics—Family relationships. 2. Epilepsy—Psychological
aspects. 3. Epilepsy—Social aspects. I. Title.
RC372.L383   1999
362.1'96853—dc21   98-42636

Contents

Epilepsy
and the Family

A NEW GUIDE

Chapter One

Epilepsy:
Its Characteristics
and Impact

Patrick was interested in a career in medicine because his father had epilepsy. Although the seizures frightened him at first, he quickly learned how to help his father when an attack occurred. Rather than running about excitedly and calling for help, he would safeguard his father, piling pillows around him and moving objects that might injure the convulsing man. He would advise friends and relatives what to do and what not to do during attacks. If young children were present, he would reassure them that the seizure was frightening but not dangerous. His father admitted that he relied heavily upon his son, and that without Patrick's keen sense of when a seizure was about to occur he would have suffered many more injuries than he did. Patrick was 3 years old at the time.

Miriam's young son, David, had had seizures since birth and had undergone several operations to treat birth defects associated with the epilepsy. Even with his mother's constant attention, David had as many as fifteen seizures a day. Miriam was obsessed with the dangers that he faced every time he had a seizure. Her husband understood her preoccupation with David and spent all his spare time helping with his supervision and medications. Even so, the child took up all of Miriam's time and attention. Their four other children had to look after themselves.

Elizabeth married a man who had his first seizure a few days before the wedding. The epilepsy soon became intractable despite a variety of medications and other less conventional treatments. Elizabeth's every action had to take her husband's seizure disorder into account. Her thorough preoccupation with it became clear when she went to renew her driver's license. Looking at the form she had filled out, the clerk asked her to answer additional questions about her epilepsy. After a moment of confusion she realized that she had indicated on the form that she suffered from epilepsy. Even after the error was pointed out to her, Elizabeth felt that her answer was quite accurate: her husband's seizures were as much an impairment for her as for him.

Epilepsy is a tendency to have recurrent seizures. Seizures are episodes of disorganized electrical activity in the brain that can produce a broad spectrum of signs and symptoms, ranging from involuntary movements to loss of consciousness (see Table 1). Like any chronic medical problem, epilepsy affects not only the person suffering from it but also that person's family. Parents whose children develop epilepsy must cope with special restrictions, constant medications, and perhaps learning or behavior disorders. Other children in the family may be deprived of their fair share of attention because of the extra demands of the child with seizures. A wife may find that after her husband develops epilepsy he can no longer support the family or loses interest in sex. Alternatively, for some people with epilepsy, seizures are fully controlled with medications and minor adjustments to lifestyle. Whether the impact of the seizure disorder is highly intrusive or minimally disruptive to any family is often determined as much by the

TABLE 1
Characteristics of Seizures and Epilepsy

Seizures	Epilepsy
Caused by inappropriate electrical activity in the brain	Characterized by recurrent seizures or a neurologic syndrome associated with seizures
Neurologic signs and symptoms are transient	Seizures occur with little or no provocation
Altered consciousness, involuntary movements, and disturbed perceptions often occur	One or multiple seizure types may occur, and seizures may change with age
Defined by neurologic signs and symptoms and EEG patterns	Defined by spectrum of seizure types, EEG patterns, and clinical setting

family's techniques for dealing with the disorder as by the volatility of the disorder itself.

The impact of epilepsy on a particular family is partly determined by the type and frequency of the seizures. Even well-controlled epilepsy, in which the affected person hardly ever has a seizure, can be very disruptive. The threat of seizures, even when seizures have been under control for many years, can inhibit the activities of the individual and the family. That a family member has a seizure disorder remains a major consideration in the family's plans and activities. Parents may obsessively shelter their affected child. The husband of a woman who has only occasional seizures may doubt that she can be relied upon in a crisis. The entire family may treat the person with epilepsy as "sick" even decades after the last seizure has occurred.

If the seizures are poorly controlled and the affected person has frequent and unpredictable seizures, they can destabilize the family and drain its financial and emotional resources. Circumstances thought to precipitate seizures take on an almost magical significance, and the family will go to great lengths to avoid them. If social activities seem to bring on a young girl's seizures, her parents may isolate her from friends. A couple may decide not to have a second child because the wife had more frequent seizures during her first pregnancy. Many families fear that any change in lifestyle or routine, however slight, may trigger a new round of seizures. Family interactions can become desperately rigid and oppressive. The person with seizures may be surrounded by tension even if all members of the family insist that the epilepsy is not a significant problem.

In the final analysis, the goal for every person with epilepsy is to lead as normal a life as possible. Ideally this is a life without seizures; if that cannot be achieved, it is at least a life free of unreasonable fears or prohibitions. The family helps to determine what kind of life the person with epilepsy will live. Lowered expectations can become self-fulfilling prophecies. An adult who is expected to take little responsibility within the family because of a seizure disorder often lives up to that expectation. An overprotected child will grow up to be an unprepared adult. A person who has always been treated as "sick" will have trouble realizing her own capabilities. In fact, most people with seizures are able to lead largely normal lives. Informed and understanding families are vitally important in helping them do so.

Characteristics of Epilepsy

Epilepsy occurs in men, women, and children of every culture and nationality. In the United States it affects at least one out of every two hundred people. It is a disturbance of the electrical activity of the brain that can abruptly interfere with behavior, perception, movement, consciousness, or other brain functions. Individual attacks of disorganized electrical activity are called seizures; when attacks occur repeatedly, the problem is called a seizure disorder or epilepsy. Because of the stigma attached to the term epilepsy, some physicians avoid using it. Patients may be told instead that they have seizures, fits, brain attacks, convulsions, drop attacks, or other problems that do not include the terms epilepsy or epileptic.

The term "convulsion" is usually reserved for seizures in which jerking of the limbs or trunk and loss of conscious ness are prominent features. Seizures are so often referred to as convulsions that physicians routinely call medications to suppress seizures "anticonvulsants," but a more accurate term is antiepileptic medications. It is a bit misleading to call antiepileptic medications anticonvulsants, since these medications are used for all types of seizures, not just for convulsions.

Inappropriate, disorganized, or excessive electrical activity in the brain is believed to be the common element in all seizure disorders. Different types of seizures may have little else in common besides this electrical dysfunction. Nerve cells in the brain communicate and regulate one another's activities primarily by way of electrical signals running along fine extensions from the body of one nerve cell, or neuron, to other neurons (Figure 1). Seizures occur when this electrical activity runs amok and the exchange between nerve cells becomes chaotic. Seizures seem to be an especially likely consequence of this electrical chaos when the nerve cells in the most superficial layers of the brain are involved. Coordinated or at least somewhat disciplined activity in this part of the brain is essential for normal consciousness, sensation, strength, and movement. During a seizure, one or all of these brain functions may be affected to varying degrees.

In some types of epilepsy, seizures cause loss of consciousness, whereas in others, consciousness is minimally impaired if at all. Some types of seizures invariably include involuntary movement and hallucinations, and others never produce abnormal movements or changes in vision, hearing, smell, taste, or other sensations. Although there are many different types of epilepsy, most people with seizure disorders experience only one type of seizure.

Misconceptions and misunderstandings develop at least in part because epilepsy is not a single entity with simple characteristics, and seizures are not a single phenomenon with stereotypical features. Carl, a businessman who developed seizures after a head injury, insisted for several years that he did not have epilepsy because his episodes of altered consciousness involved wandering, peculiar movements and behavior,

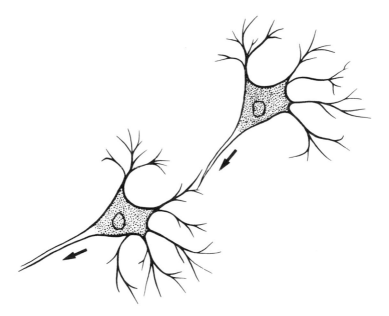

FIGURE 1.   Schematic drawing of nerve cells (neurons). Electrical signals travel along projections (dendrites and axons) to and from nerve cells to transmit information from one part of the brain to another. The brain has billions of cells forming complex circuits. The message traveling from one cell to another may either inhibit or excite the nerve cell receiving the signal.

and temporary loss of memory but no jerking of his arms or legs. He insisted that a person with epilepsy always lost consciousness, fell down, and had convulsive movements of the limbs. What Carl recognized as epilepsy—and what many nonmedical people consider to be epilepsy—is a generalized tonic-clonic, or so-called grand mal, seizure. The type of seizure he was experiencing is a partial seizure with complex symptoms, also known as a complex partial or psychomotor seizure. This common misconception about seizures and epilepsy allowed Carl to deny having a condition that he associated with mental deficiency. He preferred to believe that his peculiar behavior and memory loss were symptoms of an emotional or psychological disorder. Some physicians hearing of his problem were inclined to agree with him, a complicity based on the difficulty in distinguishing some types of seizures from psychiatric phenomena.

Carl's denial that he had epilepsy is a common response, but there is no way to anticipate how any individual will react to the diagnosis of epilepsy. Marianne, a 25-year-old medical technician with transient episodes of numbness on one side of her body, was relieved to discover that her problem was an unusual type of seizure disorder called focal sensory seizures. She had feared that the peculiar sensations were evidence of a mental illness; and, unlike the businessman, Marianne found the prospect of "going crazy" much more terrifying than having seizures.

Although seizure disorders come in many different types, some features occur with striking frequency, and some attacks appear remarkably similar in many different people. Recurring features in different individuals form the basis for classifying seizure types (Table 2). Classification is useful because it provides a basis for choosing effective therapies. Some types of seizures, such as generalized absence seizures of childhood (also called petit mal or generalized nonconvulsive), are remarkably consistent from person to person. This makes them relatively easy to identify and simplifies the choice of

TABLE 2
Types of Seizures

Generalized	Partial
Convulsive	Simple
Nonconvulsive	Complex

treatment. Other seizure types are quite variable from individual to individual, although the seizure experienced by any one person is likely to have similar features each time it recurs. Complex partial seizures occur at any age, are extremely diverse in character, and consequently may be very difficult to identify in their least common forms. Deciding what specific form of seizures a person has may not be at all simple, but making an accurate diagnosis is worth the effort because the diagnosis in large part dictates the therapy, determines the outlook, and provides insight into the problems likely to be faced by the affected person and his family.

Provocative Stimuli and Seizure Thresholds

Epilepsy by definition involves recurrent seizures or at least the risk of recurrent seizures. A person who has had only one seizure does not necessarily have epilepsy. An isolated seizure may be nothing more than a one-time response to a head injury, nervous system infection, or chemical imbalance (such as low blood sugar, low levels of calcium or magnesium, or drug overdose). After recovering from these conditions, the person may be at no greater risk of seizures than people in the general population. Even a person who has had two or more seizures that were provoked by a stimulus likely to produce seizures in anyone, such as a high-voltage electric shock, does not have epilepsy. Women with complicated pregnancies that result in high blood pressure and kidney disturbances may have seizures—a condition called toxemia of pregnancy or eclampsia—but these women would not be described as having epilepsy. They might have seizures each time they develop eclampsia, and they might develop eclampsia each time they get pregnant, but the seizures are attributable to a temporary condition, and after it ends their risk of seizures falls back to normal. Therefore they do not have epilepsy.

But what is a "normal" risk of seizures? Any person, regardless of how normal his nervous system is, can be stressed sufficiently to evoke a seizure. Severe sleep deprivation, electrical shocks, dehydration, head trauma, sunstroke, alcohol abuse, and other physical stresses can all provoke seizures in people whose brains are perfectly ordinary. How resistant we are to seizures under conditions that are known to provoke them is variable from individual to individual, but we all have a point beyond which our nervous systems cannot maintain organized activity. That is the point at which a seizure occurs.

The person with epilepsy is at risk for recurrent seizures *without* these predictably provocative stimuli. That the seizure disorder is completely controlled with medication does not change the fact that the person has epilepsy. If stopping the medication may reasonably be expected to place the person at risk of recurrent seizures, that person has epilepsy.

Epilepsy itself is not hereditary, but some nervous system disorders that cause epilepsy are inherited. In a given family, one member may have only a single seizure, and after that, if she takes medication, she may remain seizure-free for the rest of her life. We would still diagnose her as having epilepsy if we know that another member of her family has seizures. She is at higher-than-normal risk because of her personal and family history.

Sometimes a person with a family history of epilepsy will have only one seizure and then remain seizure-free for the rest of his life, even without medication. He is spared further attacks either because he is not as vulnerable to stimuli that evoke seizures as are other people in his family (in which case the label "epilepsy" may not be appropriate for him) or because he is almost never exposed to the stimuli to which they are vulnerable.

What will trigger seizures in people with epilepsy is as variable as the form the seizures may assume. Starvation, dehydration, and exhaustion may be required to provoke attacks in one person, while a single night without much sleep may provoke seizures in another person with the same type of epilepsy. In most cases there is no obvious explanation for the difference. Even closely related people whose heredity makes them seizure-prone may require dramatically different conditions for seizures to occur. One child with generalized tonic-clonic seizures that develop only after several days of sleep deprivation may have a brother whose seizures occur whenever he sees flashing lights.

Sleeplessness, physical exhaustion, trauma, infection, and alcohol abuse are common precipitants of seizures in people whose epilepsy had been well-controlled previously. But the most common reason for recurrent seizures is failure to take one's antiepileptic drugs as prescribed (Table 3). All of these provocative stimuli and situations must be avoided to minimize the risk of seizures. For most people this means developing daily routines that eliminate irregular hours and excessive burdens and that ensure that one does not skip medications. It is also important to pay extra attention to health issues and personal hygiene. Dental problems, foot infections, colds, and other common illnesses can rapidly escalate from minor annoyances to major health threats by evoking seizures.

In fact, in a person with epilepsy, an increase in seizures may be the first sign of another unrecognized health problem. For example, nighttime (nocturnal) seizures may be the first indication of a gum infection. Uncontrollable seizures that disappear when the patient is admitted to the hospital for closer observation may indicate well-concealed alcohol

TABLE 3
Stimuli That Can Provoke Seizures

Missing doses of medication

Sleep deprivation

Trauma

Alcohol withdrawal

Barbiturate withdrawal

Amphetamine abuse

Flashing lights

abuse. Abuse of other drugs, such as cocaine, amphetamines, phencyclidine (PCP), and barbiturates, may also trigger seizures. Nevertheless, the hallmark of epilepsy is the predisposition to recurrent *unprovoked* seizures; the search for a cause of each seizure is usually fruitless.

Some women with seizures notice an increase in episodes around the time of menstruation. These are called catamenial seizures and are assumed to be triggered by hormonal fluctuations. The hormonal changes of the menstrual cycle are not avoidable, but adjusting a woman's dose of antiepileptic medication or adding another medication at specific points in the cycle may keep her free of seizures. Such fine adjustments in medication usually become unnecessary after menopause.

Much less common, but potentially more problematic, are so-called reflex epilepsies, in which seizures may be triggered by nothing more than a specific noise, sight, action, or even thought. As routine and unavoidable an activity as eating initiates seizures in some people. Roger, a young man with posttraumatic complex partial seizures, developed a generalized convulsion whenever he looked to the left if he did not turn his head while shifting his eyes. In time, most people learn what will trigger their seizures and try to avoid it. Unfortunately, in rare cases the provocative stimulus is an activity, such as sexual intercourse, which, if avoided, can have far-reaching consequences.

A person who is vulnerable to seizures is said to have a lowered seizure threshold. The threshold may be temporarily lowered, so that just one seizure occurs in a lifetime, or it may be chronically lowered, resulting in a tendency to have recurrent seizures under conditions that provoke no seizures in most of the healthy population. Certain structural and chemical abnormalities in the brain will predictably lower the seizure threshold. A brain tumor, a malformation of blood vessels in the head, or a central nervous system infection will typically increase susceptibility to seizures. A seizure may also occur after head injury in an automobile accident or after brain damage from a stroke. In either case the increased susceptibility to seizures may be very brief or may become permanent.

Epilepsy may be the first sign of a problem, but seizures do not necessarily occur with all injuries to the nervous system, even if the nervous system damage is persistent and substantial. For example, Harry, who was diagnosed with tuberous sclerosis—a hereditary disease causing abnormalities in the brain, skin, and other organs—had only minor skin changes and was a successful mathematician and university professor. But his infant son suffered from severe mental retardation and uncontrollable seizures. The effects of hereditary diseases can vary tremendously from one family member to another. Often the nonseizure consequences of a congenital or hereditary problem, such as the skin changes of tuberous sclerosis, in one family member help to establish what is causing seizures in another.

If seizures can be directly linked to an underlying problem, such as a meningitis, stroke, brain contusion, or intracranial bleeding, the epilepsy is called symptomatic or secondary. When no apparent problem other than the seizures can be

TABLE 4

Differences between Idiopathic
and Symptomatic Epilepsy

Idiopathic or Primary	Symptomatic or Secondary
Brain structure is usually normal	Head trauma, meningitis, metabolic disease, stroke, or other cerebral disease is usually the underlying cause
Neurologic exam is often normal	Neurologic exam often exhibits focal deficits, dementia, partial paralysis, sensory impairment
Hereditary pattern is commonly found	Hereditary pattern is not evident, except with metabolic disease
Age of onset is predictable	Age of onset is related to the underlying cause
Seizures are usually self-limited and responsive to medication	Seizures are often unremitting and resistant to treatment
EEG is usually normal between seizures except for "markers" of seizure tendency	EEG is usually abnormal between seizures

found, or when the seizures cannot be attributed to other evident problems, the epilepsy is called idiopathic or primary (Table 4). Pediatric neurologists occasionally distinguish epilepsy with neither an apparent cause nor a familial pattern from epilepsy with no apparent cause but a suspected familial or hereditary pattern. The former may be referred to as cryptogenic and the latter as idiopathic. Both cryptogenic and idiopathic are terms traditionally used to indicate that the cause of the problem is unknown. People with idiopathic epilepsy are assumed to have subtle, genetically based abnormalities in the structure or function of the brain that are beyond the resolution of available investigative techniques. Distinguishing between symptomatic and idiopathic or cryptogenic epilepsy is important in defining the probable course (prognosis) of the disorder and in choosing an appropriate therapy to manage it.

Epilepsy as a Chronic Disease

Many of the problems that develop with epilepsy also occur with other chronic health problems, but epilepsy poses special problems, both for persons who have the disorder and for those who are intimately involved with them. Much of the disruptiveness associated with epilepsy comes from its unpredictability. It is more often a threat than an active condition. Unlike chronic heart, liver, kidney, or lung disease, it does not follow a relatively consistent pattern that can be used to predict incidents and to make long-term or even short-term plans. Decisions about schooling, work, marriage, and reproduction are confounded by this unpredictability. Even though epilepsy is rarely lethal or even progressively debilitating, it is often sufficiently erratic to frustrate even the most determined individual. The inhibition provoked by having a seizure disorder may be more limiting than any disability caused by the seizures themselves, which are transient.

The need to take one or several medications every day is as much a nuisance with epilepsy as it is with any chronic condition, but the advantages are much less obvious than those associated with taking a drug for congestive heart failure, asthma, or arthritis. A person with chest pain and limited exercise tolerance can recognize immediately the benefit of taking medications. With epilepsy, seizure control is never certain, even with an ideal dose of antiepileptic medication, and any side effects of the medications—lethargy, stomach upset, hair loss, weight gain, gum problems, or rash—are usually very obvious. The person with epilepsy is hard-pressed to continue taking medications that cause these discomforts without completely controlling seizures. Assurances that the situation would be much worse without the treatment are not always sufficient to induce the person to take antiepileptic drugs.

Although perfect seizure control is elusive for many people, more than 80 percent of people with seizures will be well-controlled on antiepileptic medications. Ironically, the person most likely to discontinue the medication is the one with the best result. People free of seizures for months or years are not always inclined to continue taking medications for a problem they no longer experience on a daily basis—although for many other people with epilepsy, the fear of losing this control is a strong motivator. If seizures are not well-controlled, people may simply give up on the medication in an effort to shed the "sick role" that epilepsy forced upon them. Obviously, this behavior is self-defeating, since they just become sicker and more dependent as their seizures increase. The family's tendency to give the affected member special consideration and to lower expectations for him is reinforced by this self-defeating behavior.

Complicating the life of the person with seizures is the need to explain involuntary behaviors (Table 5). During complex partial seizures, some people make peculiar noises, defecate while still dressed, undress in public, or obsessively drink water. When they regain full consciousness, they are perplexed or embarrassed by the socially inappropriate behavior they exhibited. Compounding the problem is the reluctance of people witnessing the peculiar behavior to accept it as involuntary, because it seems so purposeful. Even if the person exhibiting the disturbed behavior is known to have seizures, family and colleagues are often inclined to suspect that the behavior was in some way intentional, especially if the behavior is destructive or disabling. Unsympathetic or skeptical family and colleagues may expect or demand justification for involuntary behavior long after it has been firmly linked to epilepsy.

TABLE 5

Common Initial Signs of Epilepsy

Staring spells
Bedwetting
Memory gaps
Wandering
Tongue-biting during sleep
Violent muscle spasms during sleep

Common Misconceptions

Less than fifty years ago a British medical journal indicated that the general public believed people with epilepsy were "mentally imbalanced, dull, or frankly mentally defective, liable to progressive mental deterioration, awkward to live with, antisocial or potentially criminal, incurable . . . unemployable, and persons who should be sequestered in institutions." These notions are less pervasive today, but highly publicized criminal cases that use an "epilepsy defense," and tenuous disability claims based on epilepsy, have done nothing to improve the image of people with seizure disorders that is generally held by the public. In nonmedical circles, epilepsy is still viewed as a hereditary problem and often considered a type of mental illness.

Family members and employers sometimes worry that violent behavior will occur with seizures. Mood swings and phenomena associated with mood swings, such as shouting, crying, or laughing, may occur during seizures but are never the basis for purposeful acts. The view that a burglary or a murder may be perpetrated during a seizure is ludicrous. Certainly some people who are criminals also have epilepsy, but premeditated or even complex goal-directed behavior producing a criminal outcome is impossible during a seizure.

Another common misconception is that seizures and brain damage inevitably occur together. This view probably survives because people with severe brain damage often do develop seizures. This does not mean that everyone with epilepsy has brain damage or even that epilepsy is a sign of brain damage. With idiopathic epilepsy, structural brain damage or anomalies are relatively rare and mental impairment is generally not present.

Although people with seizures soon recognize that these stereotypes are baseless, they also realize that it is to their advantage to conceal their disorder. Even the most enlightened employers will choose a person without epilepsy over a person with epilepsy, if other factors are equal. Attempting to convince friends and employers that seizures do not indicate a mental or emotional defect often exposes the person with epilepsy to further sanctions for frankness.

The Struggle to Conceal Epilepsy

Simply being labeled as epileptic can cause considerable social damage. Once a person is recognized as having seizures, she loses many privileges. Some losses, such as having her driver's license revoked after a seizure, are legally mandated and are defensible on safety grounds. Others are less justifiable and have broader implications. Life insurance becomes more difficult to secure, and health insurance is often more expensive. Marital choices become more restricted and employment opportunities more limited. Almost 20 percent of parents whose children do not have seizures admit to being opposed to the idea of their children marrying someone with epilepsy. The number of parents who actually oppose it but would not admit this bias in an opinion survey is probably much higher.

Among people with epilepsy whose employers know their diagnosis, about 40 percent have problems securing or retaining jobs. What makes the epilepsy known by employers is not merely seizures on the job or absences caused by poor seizure control; more often it is an admission on an allegedly confidential health questionnaire or questions raised by medications taken on the job. In an era of self-insured corporations and closely aligned managed care associations, confidentiality has become a scarce commodity, routinely guaranteed but rarely provided.

People with low seizure thresholds may risk recurrent seizures by not taking their medications at the prescribed times if taking the medication would raise questions. Anita, a young woman with well-controlled and well-concealed seizures, was advised by her physician not to drink alcohol because of the possible interaction with her antiepileptic medication. After four years of compliance with these instructions, she abruptly stopped her medications. Her friends had questioned why she never consumed any alcohol, not even social drinks. Rather than reveal her medical condition or lie, Anita chose to neutralize the growing suspicions of her friends and colleagues by agreeing to join them for beers. She felt obliged to heed her physician's advice, however, and so she stopped taking the antiepileptic medication when she started drinking socially. Then, to avoid being reprimanded by her physician for not taking her medicine, she stopped going to her doctor. Acceptance by one's peers is as powerful a motivator for people with epilepsy as it is for people without epilepsy.

Many young adults conceal their epilepsy to avoid rejection by potential spouses. As marriage becomes likely, revealing the neurologic problem is even more difficult. If a seizure occurs during the engagement or shortly after the marriage, the uninformed partner is likely to feel duped or at least untrusted. If the disillusioned partner subsequently abandons the person with epilepsy, it may be because the deception undermined the relationship, and not because the epilepsy itself was unacceptable.

The most common setting for concealment of epilepsy is the

workplace. Curiously, people involved in manual labor are more likely to notify employers of their neurologic problem than those working in managerial or white-collar positions. An executive with epilepsy faces more resistance to advancement than a carpenter with the same disorder, even though the carpenter runs a much higher risk of an on-the-job mishap related to seizures. Presumably the common misconception that thinking cannot be completely normal in someone with epilepsy interferes with an executive's advancement, whereas skill at manual tasks is routinely perceived as less dependent on intellectual discipline. Also, for the sake of his own safety, a construction worker might want his boss to know the risks of certain tasks.

Types of Seizures

Accurately identifying the type or cause of epilepsy is the first step in treating the disorder. If an underlying condition, such as a nervous system infection or a tumor, is responsible for the seizures, it must be eliminated or managed as part of the treatment. Even if no basis for the epilepsy can be found, the seizures can usually be treated and controlled if the drugs used are appropriate for the type of seizure. In fact, the majority of seizure disorders remain unexplained even after extensive investigation. As with any diagnosis, the conclusion that the seizures are not symptomatic of an injury to the brain or a metabolic problem is nothing more than the best guess that can be made based on the information available. The cause of an idiopathic epilepsy may become apparent long after the initial evaluation. A slow-growing tumor may produce nothing more than seizures for years; a metabolic disease involving the brain may cause seizures initially and mental impairment years later. Fortunately, these insidious problems are rarely the explanation for an idiopathic seizure disorder. Most seizure disorders that cannot be explained after routine neurologic tests remain unexplained for the rest of the person's life.

Identifying the type of seizure provides valuable information to the physician, patient, and family. Children with generalized absence (petit mal) seizures have problems and prognoses very different from those of children with complex partial seizures, even though both groups of children may have little more than staring spells as evidence of the epilepsy. The treatment and inconvenience of complex partial (psychomotor) seizures in adults are distinct from those of generalized tonic-clonic (grand mal) seizures, even though both are routinely associated with profoundly altered consciousness.

Several features of a person's seizure disorder determine what type of seizure the person has. Age at onset of the seizures, the area of the brain that is most disturbed by abnormal electrical activity, the sequence of physical and mental changes that occur during the seizure, and the pattern of electroencephalographic (EEG or brain wave) recordings during the seizure all enter into the classification of the seizure type. In many cases, a full and accurate description of the symptoms and signs before, during, and after the acute attack provides enough information for the physician to identify the seizure disorder.

Unfortunately, the reports of the patient and of families or friends witnessing the attacks are usually incomplete or inaccurate. The patient is often confused or unconscious during the seizure, and relatives and friends are invariably frightened and upset. Brain wave changes associated with a seizure are much more objective, but obtaining a recording before, during, and after an episode is difficult, if not impossible, with people who have infrequent seizures. Because of this, the physician's initial impression of the type of seizure may need to be revised as more information about the episodes becomes available.

Most seizure types can be defined as either generalized or

TABLE 6
Types of Seizures

Proper Name	Common Name
Generalized seizures	
Tonic-clonic or convulsive	Grand mal
Clonic	
Tonic	
Absence or nonconvulsive*	Petit mal, absence
Infantile spasms*	
Atonic and akinetic*	Drop attacks
Myoclonic*	
Partial seizures	
Simple motor	Focal motor, jacksonian
Simple somatosensory	Focal sensory
Simple special sensory	
Simple autonomic	
Simple psychic-cognitive	
Complex	Psychomotor, temporal lobe
Secondarily generalized	

* Also called minor motor seizures

partial (Table 6). With generalized seizures, both sides of the brain seem to be disturbed simultaneously by abnormal electrical activity. In partial seizures, a local abnormality stays limited to part of the brain or spreads to involve both sides of the brain (Figure 2). Every seizure, whether generalized or partial, has several discrete stages, which are especially obvious in the case of complex partial seizures. The stage with the most dramatic electrical disorganization is called the *ictus* of the seizure. This is often preceded by some type of warning, called the *aura*. The aura is actually part of the seizure proper, even though most people perceive it as a distinct phenomenon. The minutes or hours of abnormal consciousness following the seizure are called the *postictal period*. The interval between seizures is the *interictal period*.

Generalized Seizures

The person with generalized seizures will lose consciousness for seconds or minutes, a lapse sometimes more obvious to others than to the affected person. The most common types of generalized seizures are the tonic-clonic (or grand mal) and absence (or petit mal) forms.

Generalized Tonic-Clonic Seizures
(Convulsive, Grand Mal Seizures)

Generalized convulsive (grand mal) seizures can develop at any age. The affected person has an abrupt loss of consciousness followed by convulsive movements of the body. These convulsive movements are called tonic-clonic because there are two phases of muscle activity, one in which limb and

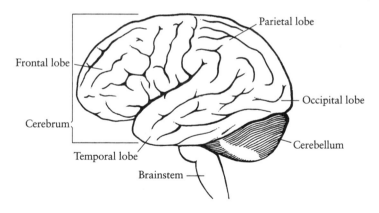

FIGURE 2. Principal divisions of the brain. The cerebrum is the part of the brain most disturbed when a seizure occurs. The most superficial layers of nerve cells in the cerebrum are called the cortex. The cerebellum is primarily responsible for the coordination of movements. Information from the brain travels to different parts of the body through the brainstem and the spinal cord. The spinal cord is an extension of the brainstem. All of the structures indicated on this diagram are inside the skull.

trunk muscles become extremely rigid as they persistently, or tonically, enter a violent spasm of contraction, and one in which the muscles contract rhythmically, that is, clonically. In the tonic phase the person may arch his back or forcefully keep his arms and legs parallel to his trunk. Changes in breathing may be obvious and may produce gasping noises and a bluish complexion. These changes give the false impression that the seizure victim is suffocating. Such worrisome signs routinely pass in a matter of seconds, and skin color returns to normal. In the clonic phase the limbs and trunk jerk or thrash about as muscle contractions become rhythmic and intermittent. The contractions typically slow down before stopping after about a minute. This type of seizure is usually called a convulsion (Table 7).

Tongue biting and urination often occur during grand mal seizures. Even when the tongue is not bitten, the gums or cheek may suffer minor cuts from involuntary jaw movements. The person may also defecate or forcefully kick nearby objects. Violent contractions of the muscles about the shoulder may dislocate the arm at the shoulder joint. Elderly people occasionally develop spine fractures from the force of spinal muscle contractions, but most people with this type of seizure do not hurt themselves unless they suffer an injury during the initial collapse.

These attacks appear with little or no warning. If there is a warning, it is usually just a few seconds of malaise or lightheadedness preceding the episode. The acute (ictal) seizure phenomena last several seconds to a few minutes. Subsequently, the person will be poorly responsive to all stimuli for minutes or hours (the postictal period).

If this type of seizure occurs while the person with epilepsy is sleeping, he may wonder why his tongue is sore or why there is urine in his bed, but he may not realize that he had a seizure. Sometimes the person can recall a momentary sense of paralysis and panic, a flash of light, or distortion of sounds, but that is all he remembers of the event. Children who de-

TABLE 7

Features of Generalized Tonic-Clonic
Seizures (Grand Mal)

Little or no warning of impending seizure

EEG diffusely abnormal at start

Loss of posture with high risk of injury

Loss of consciousness

Loss of bladder or bowel control likely

Violent contraction of limb and trunk muscles

Confusion lasting minutes afterward

velop seizures during sleep may be punished for bedwetting or
be referred for psychiatric evaluation before a seizure disorder
is recognized. An adult's bed partner may be kicked during
the clonic phase of the seizure and stop sleeping in the same
bed with the person with epilepsy because of what is interpreted as restlessness.

Most people do not grow out of this type of seizure disorder. That is, simply growing older does not improve one's
chances of remission, nor does the character of the seizure
usually change with age. Seizures may be inapparent for years
and then recur for no obvious reason. Fortunately, antiepileptic drugs are usually effective in suppressing the convulsions in most people with exclusively this type of seizure disorder.

Generalized Absence Seizures (Petit Mal Seizures or Absence Attacks)

The person with generalized absence epilepsy is usually a
child, and the principal feature of the seizure disorder is a momentary loss of consciousness (Table 8). Seizures usually appear at 6 to 12 years of age and disappear or change to an-

TABLE 8

Features of Generalized Absence Seizures (Petit Mal)

No warning of impending seizure
EEG shows typical 3/sec spike-and-slow-wave pattern
No loss of posture
Loss of consciousness
No loss of bladder or bowel control
No violent limb or trunk movements
No confusion afterward

other type by the end of adolescence. The seizures may not be recognized for years because the child's absence attacks may not be thought to be anything more than peculiar behavior. The child abruptly becomes inattentive and may stop talking in the middle of a sentence without even realizing the interruption in speech has occurred. During the seizures, these children do not fall down, jerk their limbs, or thrash about. They may blink or make other subtle facial movements, but more characteristic is an interruption of any movements that were occurring. A child who is sitting or standing when the attack occurs remains sitting or standing. The brain wave pattern in children with this type of epilepsy is very helpful in establishing the diagnosis (Figure 3).

Transient loss of consciousness, the principal manifestation of absence seizures, is also a common feature of complex partial seizures. When absence seizures are responsible for the absence attacks, the return to normal consciousness is just as abrupt as the loss of consciousness. There is usually no confusion or lethargy following the seizure. The child may not even realize that he or she had an episode of altered consciousness.

When complex partial seizures are responsible, in contrast, the child does not abruptly return to normal consciousness but goes through a period of inattentiveness or confusion that may last minutes or hours.

Although generalized absence seizures that start in childhood usually stop in adolescence, they may persist into adult life, at which time they usually evolve into more disabling seizures. The petit mal seizures may be replaced by complex partial or grand mal seizures as the child becomes an adult. Occasionally the absence attacks persist in association with other types of seizures. Adults with no history of childhood seizures who develop staring spells do not have absence seizures but may have another type of seizure disorder, such as complex partial seizures.

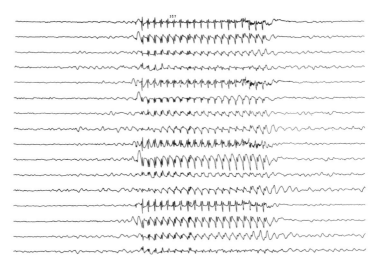

FIGURE 3. Electroencephalogram in petit mal epilepsy. The 3-per-second spike-and-slow-wave discharges that are characteristic of generalized absence (petit mal) epilepsy occupy the middle third of this 17-second recording. The child had a staring spell and was mute when these brain waves appeared.

Other Generalized Seizures

Several other types of generalized seizures are much less common than grand mal and petit mal seizures. Infants with profoundly abnormal EEGs and frequent convulsive spasms that jerk their entire bodies are said to have infantile spasms. The profoundly abnormal pattern of brain waves that persists even between apparent spasms, called hypsarrhythmia, is a sign of diffusely abnormal brain activity. Infantile spasms with hypsarrhythmia are caused by several different types of injury to the brain, but they most often develop if the child suffers trauma or inadequate oxygen (asphyxia) at birth. This type of generalized seizure disorder invariably develops between birth and 3 years of age and is usually associated with mental retardation or other obvious signs of irreversible brain damage.

Less common forms of generalized seizures include transient attacks of massive muscle jerks (myoclonic seizures) that may literally throw the affected person to the ground; diffuse body stiffening (tonic seizures); and fleeting episodes of impaired body tone (atonic attacks) that are generally seen only in children or adults with mental retardation. In each of these generalized seizure disorders a metabolic or structural problem in the brain must be carefully sought before the seizures are considered idiopathic. Myoclonic seizures, however, occur in a fairly common idiopathic syndrome called juvenile myoclonic epilepsy. In this disorder, tonic-clonic and, less commonly, absence seizures also occur.

Partial Seizures

With partial seizures, abnormal electrical activity always starts in a limited and usually discernible area of the cerebral cortex. During the seizure, the abnormal activity spreads and may even generalize to involve much of the cerebral cortex. When this happens within a few seconds, the seizure resembles a generalized tonic-clonic seizure. The only way to identify these seizures as partial (or "secondarily generalized") is to follow the spread of abnormal electrical activity on an EEG obtained during the seizure.

Partial seizures assume two basic forms: simple and complex. When the seizure consists of abnormal sensation or movement that is limited to one part of the body or disturbed perceptions involving only one sense, it is classified as a partial seizure with simple or elementary symptomatology. This is better known as a focal motor or focal sensory seizure. A partial seizure that causes changes in behavior, sensation, and movement in a variety of combinations and produces altered consciousness is generally known as a complex partial seizure.

Complex Partial Seizures (Psychomotor, Temporal Lobe Seizures)

Complex partial seizures are the most common of the partial seizures. Of all people suffering from seizures, 20 to 30 percent have this type. The first attack usually occurs at about the time of puberty, but prepubertal children and adults of all ages can also develop complex partial epilepsy. Sixty-four percent of people with complex partial seizures have at least some secondarily generalized seizures as well.

Most complex partial seizures begin in the temporal lobe on one side of the brain, and significant structural damage in the temporal lobe can be found in some people. But for most, no obvious structural problem responsible for the seizures is discovered. Even in these cases, though, the focus of epileptic activity is usually in the temporal lobe, and therefore these seizures are also called temporal lobe seizures. This is a misleading name, in that abnormal electrical activity arising in the temporal lobe can produce other kinds of seizures besides complex partial seizures, and some complex partial seizures begin outside the temporal lobe. Nevertheless, temporal lobe

TABLE 9
Features of Complex Partial Seizures
(Psychomotor or Temporal Lobe)

Aura often warns of impending seizures
EEG shows abnormality starting locally
Loss of posture may occur
Altered or loss of consciousness may occur
Abnormal limb movements may occur
Emotional or thought disorder may be prominent
Confusion persists for minutes or hours afterward

seizure disorder is a very old term, and, like grand mal and petit mal, it is still widely used.

Complex partial seizures are often difficult to recognize because of the variety of abnormal behaviors shown by people with this disorder (Table 9). This variability may lead friends, family members, and even physicians to suspect a psychological basis for much, if not all, of the abnormal behavior observed. Some people with complex partial seizures do have psychiatric problems distinct from their seizure disorders, but most do not.

The aura
Automatic behavior or peculiar sensations often precede complex partial seizures and occur even though the person is alert (Table 10). During this stage of the seizure (the aura), the affected person may abruptly feel compelled to make some type of movement, such as turning his head to the right or left or demanding, pouring, or drinking water. Chewing movements, lip-smacking, spitting, or grimacing are part of the aura for

TABLE 10

Common Auras with Complex Partial Seizures

Upset stomach or nausea

Urgent need to defecate

Unpleasant smells or tastes

Auditory or visual hallucinations

Automatic behavior sequences

Depersonalization

Intense fear

Déjà vu

Jamais vu

some people, although these automatic movements also may appear during the seizure proper. Often a person with complex partial seizures will recognize some familiar smell, movement, or premonition and may announce that he is going to have a seizure.

With the *uncinate* form of complex partial seizures, the person senses and often complains of a disagreeable smell or taste. The name refers to the uncus of the temporal lobe, a part of the brain which was once considered important in the perception of odors. Complaints of nausea and abdominal cramps are fairly common in uncinate seizures and may lead to vomiting, sweating, and pallor.

Auditory hallucinations also occur in some auras. These usually consist of music or a buzzing sound, but occasionally they are more menacing and involve threatening voices. Similar phenomena are an early sign of psychotic disturbances, such as schizophrenia, and may cause delays in diagnosis and treatment as these alternative diagnoses are pursued. Visual hallucinations occur less frequently than auditory hallucinations. Even less common—but sometimes reported—are feelings of depersonalization and paranoid ideas. With depersonalization, the person feels separated from his body. Victims of this delusion feel as if they are watching their soulless bodies go through activities in which they are not involved. Other delusional complaints include feelings that they are being persecuted by friends, family, and strangers and that remarks and activities occurring around them are actually referring to them. The person may feel that all the world is involved in a conspiracy against him. More common are attacks of intense, groundless fear. Any of these psychiatric symptoms may contribute to these patients' occasionally being misdiagnosed as schizophrenic, but persecutory auditory hallucinations are most likely to lead to this misdiagnosis. The duration of epileptic hallucinations is seconds to minutes—much shorter than the usual schizophrenic hallucinations.

Also characteristic of some complex partial auras are feelings of intense familiarity with events just occurring (déjà vu) or total unfamiliarity with events that have occurred many times before (jamais vu). These are not abnormal feelings—many people without neurologic problems experience them from time to time—but their association with seizures makes them helpful indicators of an impending seizure in some people.

Abnormal electrical discharges detected by EEG may be just as prominent during the aura as during the seizure proper, but the person having a seizure perceives the two stages quite differently. He can usually describe the aura vividly and in considerable detail, even while it is occurring. After the seizure is over, the affected person usually remembers the aura but has no memory of the ictus. Occasionally the aura occurs without any other seizure activity. This simply means that the spread of abnormal electrical activity has not followed the pattern of a conventional attack. Auras occur with other partial or generalized seizures, but they are most complex with complex partial (psychomotor) seizures.

The ictus

The seizure proper or ictus in complex partial seizures may be just a prolonged staring spell or may evolve into a generalized tonic-clonic (grand mal) seizure. Fairly complicated but pointless behavior such as running, laughing, or crying may occur. Most common are lip-smacking, swallowing, or picking or rubbing with one's hands. The person may wander aimlessly, speak in unintelligible phrases, drink water, go to the bathroom to urinate or defecate, or simply hide. Rarely, patients appear to have sexual climax during the seizure; this phenomenon is most common in patients with seizures triggered by sexual excitement.

During the ictus, which lasts seconds or minutes, the person with complex partial seizures loses consciousness or has a profoundly altered state of consciousness. He will remember little or none of the episode when he has recovered from the seizure. The ictus is usually not associated with incontinence, tongue-biting, or muscle-jerking unless the episode progresses to a generalized tonic-clonic seizure. With especially brief seizures, the person may be completely unaware that a seizure has occurred. These absence attacks resemble generalized absence (petit mal) seizures, but the EEG will not show the typical pattern of petit mal.

The postictal period

The interval between the seizure proper and the return to normal consciousness and function lasts two to ten minutes in most cases and is characterized by disorientation, inattention, and limited activity. People with complex partial seizures that evolve into generalized seizures may become very irritable during this confused period, sometimes injuring themselves or those about them. Fortunately, postictal violence or anger is uncommon, and those few who exhibit it usually do not remember their behavior when the postictal confusion ends. This behavior is seen in both men and women. Rarely, people undress and act sexually provocative during the postictal period, but the behavior is easily recognized as purposeless.

The interictal state

The interval between unequivocal seizure episodes is called the interictal period. At least in some people with complex partial seizures, psychologic problems may be obvious even during the interictal period, when they are free of seizures. After years of seizures, personality traits and psychologic disturbances of the interictal period that were not evident before or soon after the appearance of the seizure disorder may become very disruptive for the affected person and his family. These interictal complications are considered in detail in the next chapter and in Chapter 9.

Focal Motor, Focal Sensory, and Jacksonian Seizures

Focal seizures are partial seizures that affect movement or sensation in a limited area of the body. Evidence of the seizure may be nothing more than recurrent numbness in an arm or jerking of a leg (Table 11). If the abnormality is this limited, the person is said to have focal motor or focal sensory seizures, and the symptoms occurring are called simple or elementary. During these simple partial seizures, the person usually remains relatively alert, while part of a limb or an entire limb, or even one entire side of the body, has rhythmic involuntary contractions. Some focal sensory seizures involve vision or hearing. With this type of epilepsy the affected person may have transient episodes of peculiar vision or hearing. Visual phenomena may involve little more than flashing lights, in which case they may be difficult to distinguish from migraine headaches (although their duration in seizures is typically briefer). Auditory complaints rarely include hearing menacing voices.

Seizures may start as simple or complex partial attacks and progress to generalized grand mal attacks. With many seizure

TABLE 11

Features of Simple Partial Seizures
(Focal Motor or Focal Sensory)

Little or no warning of impending seizures

EEG shows abnormality in a limited area

Sequential muscle contractions occur in jacksonian seizures

Focal limb movements occur in focal motor seizures

Focal numbness, burning, or tingling occurs in focal sensory seizures

No loss of consciousness

No postictal confusion

disorders the secondary generalization may occur so rapidly that the seizures appear to be generalized tonic-clonic episodes until electrical studies of the brain reveal the progressive spread of abnormal activity throughout the outer layers of the brain. If the progression occurs over seconds rather than milliseconds, the progression from a focal to a generalized seizure will be more apparent.

Twitching in the thumb may spread to the arm and lead to a generalized tonic-clonic convulsion in what is called a jacksonian "march" or jacksonian seizure (named after Hughlings Jackson, a neurologist who studied this type of sequential seizure in the nineteenth century). Simple partial seizures are especially easy to misdiagnose. Complaints of illusory flashing lights may be ascribed to eye disease, and the perception of a "crawling" or pins-and-needles sensation over an arm may be ascribed to injuries to a nerve in the affected limb. Because transient focal motor activity is often confused with a movement disorder and focal sensory activity is difficult to establish objectively, this type of seizure is often recognized only after it has been a problem for a long time. If the focal seizure becomes more generalized, the nature of the problem usually becomes obvious.

Alternatively, more progressive nervous system disorders may be misdiagnosed as partial seizures. Movement disorders are found in Huntington disease, Parkinson disease, and other degenerative diseases of the brain. The common migraine headache can give the illusion of flashing lights and other peculiar sensory phenomena. In a child, a twitching arm or facial grimace caused by Tourette syndrome may be misconstrued as focal epilepsy.

One form of focal epilepsy, called benign focal epilepsy of childhood or Rolandic epilepsy, almost always disappears as the child matures. Midtemporal central spikes, that is, spikes around the central (Rolandic) fissure of the brain, are seen on the electroencephalogram, most often during sleep. The seizures are occasionally generalized and are also most likely to occur during sleep. Muscle jerks or convulsive movements may be the only evidence of seizure activity. These seizures are easily controlled with antiepileptic drugs and stop by the end of adolescence.

The Implications of Epilepsy

Epilepsy is a group of disorders. All members of the group exhibit abnormal nerve-cell activity in the brain, but the spectrum of complaints and phenomena associated with epilepsy is enormous. What is most commonly recognized as epilepsy is the generalized tonic-clonic seizure disorder. What is most often not recognized as epilepsy is the generalized nonconvulsive or absence seizure disorder.

Regardless of what type of seizure disorder a person has, his seizures make him the victim of prejudices and misconceptions that have only recently shown signs of abating. Generalizations about the mental and emotional characteristics of people with epilepsy are inappropriate and usually inaccurate. Most types of epilepsy do not disturb the affected person's ability or desire to live and work in conventional ways. Especially in people with idiopathic epilepsy who take medication, the limitations imposed by the disorder itself may be negligible.

Chapter Two

The Adult
with Epilepsy

Personal and family problems caused by epilepsy in an adult vary from negligible to devastating. With antiepileptic treatment, many adults with epilepsy face virtually no limitations in their daily routines and of their long-term goals. The adults least affected by the disorder are those with no apparent seizures, who take their daily medications and suffer no adverse side effects. For this group, work, recreation, sexual activity, and family interactions proceed normally, largely undisturbed by the threat of seizures.

Unfortunately, this ideal is achieved infrequently. Complete control of seizures and long-term tolerance of antiepileptic medication are often elusive. Most adults with epilepsy are uncomfortably aware of their neurologic disorder, and it affects many aspects of their lives.

Social Adjustment

Adjusting to epilepsy means working, relaxing, and striving for personal goals with as much success as the average person without a seizure disorder. How well an adult copes with epilepsy is closely related to how well controlled the seizures are. Advances in treatment have been dramatic over the past few decades and promise to be equally substantial in the near future, but these developments cannot eliminate the fear and pessimism that often burden people whose seizures are poorly controlled.

The type of seizure a person has plays an important role in determining whether he can achieve a relatively normal lifestyle. The least disruptive types allow the most normal lifestyles. Social adjustment is normal in 87 percent of people with nonconvulsive absence seizures, regardless of their other problems. People with generalized tonic-clonic (grand mal) seizures that develop because of head injury, brain tumor, or encephalitis have, not surprisingly, poor social adjustments.

If problems with memory or thinking (cognitive dysfunction), personality disorders, or physical handicaps coexist with epilepsy, social adjustment is more difficult. Large studies have found that 92 percent of people whose seizures are not associated with any thought disturbances, memory deficiencies, or personality disorders lead virtually normal social lives. These people are not free of substantial problems, but the social obstacles they face are surmountable. Even in adults with epilepsy who have personality disorders—which include passive-aggressive, obsessive-compulsive, histrionic, overly dependent, narcissistic, antisocial, and paranoid behaviors—as many as 52 percent have a normal social adjustment. Cognitive dysfunction—such as impairment in the ability to reason or remember—reduces the fraction of people with epilepsy who adjust normally to 21 percent, and a combination of cognitive and personality disorders reduces that fraction to 15 percent.

An important element in the social adjustment of anyone, whether he or she has epilepsy or not, is setting reasonable goals. The physician can help both the patient and the family set realistic goals by providing an assessment of the patient's limitations and capacities. What is feasible will be determined in large part by the person's cognitive abilities, personality traits, and seizure control. An accurate appraisal of what is possible will help the person with epilepsy to realize his or her potential and will reduce family pressure to achieve unreasonable goals.

The physician can also anticipate problems and suggest strategies to circumvent them. Unfortunately, many patients consider their doctor to be just another reminder of the epilepsy, and they tend to avoid consultations. The sad result is that many manageable problems—such as impotence caused by an antiepileptic medication, mood swings as seizure control improves, and injuries suffered during seizures—may go unresolved because of the person's reticence or pessimism. But even the most concerned physician cannot supply the daily encouragement and support that people with epilepsy need. The real burden of helping a person adjust to epilepsy falls on the family.

Guilt

One of the more paradoxical adjustment problems faced by people with epilepsy is coping with guilt. Many victims of seizure disorders feel personally responsible for their predicament. This is especially true of accident victims, even when they were nothing more than innocent bystanders. "If only I'd been more careful" is a common refrain among those who have suffered head trauma leading to epilepsy. The combination of this sense of responsibility and a feeling of worthlessness caused by limitations in the person's activities can lead to depression and self-destructive behavior.

Many adults with epilepsy feel guilty about the impact their disorder has on other family members. "What will it do to my family?" was Jerry's central concern. His business career ended when his seizures began to interfere with his memory. Another man, Walter, who was already totally disabled by arthritis and heart disease, expressed the same concern even though he had no job to lose. He explained, "The kids looking at you, it upsets you." Walter's father had already had two heart attacks, and Walter was afraid that if his father saw him have a seizure, it might bring on another heart attack. The distress they have brought to their families is a common theme in discussions with people whose seizures are poorly controlled.

Family and friends inadvertently or purposefully reinforce guilt feelings when they insist that the person with epilepsy brings on the seizures by not taking appropriate measures to prevent them. The wife of a middle-aged man with idiopathic seizures that began when he was about 40 years old insisted that his seizures would not occur so often if he would eat a low-fat diet. Her admonitions were well-intentioned, but they intensified her husband's suspicion that he was to blame for the seizures that plagued him.

Aggravating these feelings of guilt is the embarrassment that comes with each epileptic attack. When the seizure occurs in public, many people feel deeply ashamed. Steve, who frequently had complex partial seizures, explained: "You sit up at night wondering if you should apologize, but you think, 'What are you apologizing for, for falling down and being sick?' I've reached the point where I don't give a damn what people think."

Being indifferent to the reactions of family, friends, and strangers is difficult, perhaps impossible. The physician often has limited contact with the person's family and friends and so has little opportunity to discuss the causes and management of the disorder with them. By involving at least the immediate family in discussions with the physician, the person with epilepsy can shift some of the burden of explanation to the doctor. Both the patient and the family must recognize that a person with seizures has no more reason to feel guilt or shame than the victim of a stroke or a heart attack.

Isolation

Whether out of embarrassment, guilt, or weariness at having to explain their seizures, people with epilepsy often withdraw from family, friends, and colleagues. All too often these groups allow or encourage this alienation because of their own discomfort with the seizure disorder. Those relationships that do not dissolve often change dramatically. Even if these surviving relationships are not fragile, the person with epilepsy routinely shelters them from anger, abuse, or even assertiveness. For example, a patient will not test her relationship with her physician unless she develops a self-destructive bent. Dependence upon a spouse may be so extreme that the person surrenders virtually all autonomy. The epileptic individuals' real or imagined loss of independence may eventually breed antagonism toward those they are dependent upon, and this anger increases their isolation from friends and colleagues.

In many cases the family isolates the epileptic member from normal family stresses out of concern that agitation will bring on a seizure. In fact, although emotional incidents may trigger seizures, they usually play a relatively minor role. Identifying situations that seem to trigger seizures is one valuable preventive measure to pursue, but attempts to eliminate emotional stress from the household environment are usually more disruptive and disturbing than the stress itself. Healthy families experience stress; trying to protect the person with epilepsy from emotional strain isolates him from the social activities and discussions that are an integral part of a normal family life.

The Sick Role

The family that designates a person with epilepsy as "sick" suspends that person's normal social responsibilities, such as providing income, assistance, and comfort to the family. In the most extreme cases, the person with seizures is not even expected to "pull himself together." A person with any illness, whether acute or chronic, typically regresses, at least temporarily, and becomes dependent upon family and friends. Unfortunately, denial of abilities, as well as of disabilities, is often part of the reaction to a neurologic disorder.

Ideally, a sick person should want to get better and should seek competent help in the struggle to recover. But sometimes a family begins to rely upon the disabilities of the person with epilepsy—whether real, contrived, or imposed—to explain family problems or to provide income from disability checks. The family may explicitly tell the person that the neurologic problem is totally disabling and that recovery is impossible even when that is far from true. The physician caring for the person designated "sick" may face considerable resentment if he considers the person with epilepsy less disabled than the family thinks he is. In such situations it may be less important to make an accurate assessment of the person's abilities and prognosis than to give the family a practical strategy for allowing the person to escape the sick role.

The physician must ascertain why the person was allowed or obliged to assume this dependent role in the first place and what purpose is served by his remaining in it. If what is needed is a steady flow of disability checks to support the family, then real work options must be found for the person or for other members of the family. If an unstable marriage is being held together by the demands of an all-consuming illness, then the instability of the marriage must be dealt with.

Rehabilitation

Life is very different after a person develops seizures, and rehabilitation is often appropriate. An executive who develops epilepsy after an automobile accident may lose both her job and her pride. A person whose entire self-image has been caught up in work may sink into a paralyzing depression if he can no longer perform his former duties. Rehabilitation must address both the realities of employment and the need for self-esteem. Getting the person involved in a group of people with similar types of seizures is often helpful. A group can dispel the feelings of isolation and hopelessness that often develop when a seizure disorder appears in adult life. Without some such intervention, the person with epilepsy is likely to become unassertive and isolated and to lose interest in work, social activities, and family life.

Return to employment should not wait for control of the seizures. People whose seizures are only partially controlled can and should work. Obviously, generalized convulsions that occur several times a day will drastically reduce a person's employability. Of the people with epilepsy who are unemployed, 70 percent have more than one seizure every six months and most have more than one seizure monthly. Only 50 percent of those who work have seizures this frequently.

It is possible that returning to some type of work may itself have an antiepileptic effect; evidence for this is the fact that employed people with seizure disorders exhibit more consistent seizure control than those who are idle. Of course, in these situations cause and effect are very difficult to disentangle.

Younger adults tend to respond better to rehabilitation programs than older people, especially if epilepsy is their only neurologic problem. Returning to work very soon after developing a seizure disorder also improves a patient's chances of becoming self-supporting. People who are on welfare or other types of financial assistance when rehabilitation begins are much less likely ever to return to work than are people who need to earn a living while undergoing rehabilitation.

Employment

One out of five adults with epilepsy believes that the greatest problem he or she faces is securing and holding a job. According to employment statistics, the outlook is not as grim as these people suspect, but anyone with a seizure disorder does face numerous employment problems. Finding and keeping a job are most difficult for those with both epilepsy and cognitive impairment, especially if the epilepsy is not fully controlled. In fact, the frequency and severity of seizures correlate best with difficulty obtaining and holding a job—a finding which suggests that real disability is a more important determinant of unemployment than social prejudice against people with epilepsy. When general unemployment levels in the economy are close to 3 or 4 percent, an adult with well-controlled seizures, a good education, and no other health problems has as good a chance of finding a job as an adult without epilepsy. Unfortunately, this is true only if the person does not mention epilepsy as a problem on the job application form.

When people with epilepsy apply for jobs, about 62 percent deny or do not mention the seizure disorder. Lying about their health status, when asked about it directly, obviously leaves these people vulnerable to dismissal if the seizure disorder is discovered after they have been on the job for days or years. This reluctance to be frank is understandable and quite reasonable, however. Of people with epilepsy who have problems securing a job, more than 40 percent are turned away simply because they admit to having epilepsy when asked about their medical history, even though 79 percent of Americans say they believe people with epilepsy should be hired for jobs that do not present special risks for them.

One very talented economist recruited to work for a European government discovered that the final application form asked specifically about epilepsy and antiepileptic medications. Although these forms were allegedly just a formality, each part of the application stated clearly that no appointment was final until the person's health status was deemed to be "satisfactory." The bulk of the medical questionnaire focused on epilepsy and mental illness. Implicit in the form was the notion that people with epilepsy and people with psychoses such as schizophrenia and manic-depression presented special risks to the government. This man's seizures were fully controlled with very little medication, but answering the questions honestly would have barred him from a job he had already been promised on the basis of his training and talent. Answering them dishonestly left him open to dismissal months or years later if the truth was discovered. Blatant and inappropriate discrimination was being practiced, but the discrimination had been legislated by the government for which he planned to work.

Of those people who do indicate on job applications that they have a seizure disorder, about 25 percent of the employable ones are unable to find work even when the employment figures for the general population are at their best. When general unemployment is high, people who tell potential employers about their epilepsy face systematic exclusion from the work force. Stephanie, a 17-year-old girl with fully controlled seizures, could not get job interviews for even the most unskilled work. Her mother investigated the problem and uncovered a consistent reluctance on the part of employers to risk hiring a young person with epilepsy. As recently as twenty years ago, only one in eight employers would hire a person who admitted to having a seizure disorder. The level of acceptance has edged up slightly over the past two decades, but epilepsy is still a formidable disadvantage in the job market.

Even people with long-standing employment are sometimes forced to retire or to accept disability leave because of their epilepsy. Of people with epilepsy who lose their jobs, about 30 percent are fired after having seizures at work. Many different types of employers force people with epilepsy out of their jobs as a matter of course. Hospital workers, law enforcement officers, and corporate managers who develop epilepsy all face pressure to give up their jobs. The concerns voiced by these employers are similar. They believe that people with epilepsy are accident-prone, that most work is too hazardous for them, that they require facilities to manage seizures on the job, and that seizures occurring on the job not only cut down on the productivity of the person with epilepsy but also disrupt the work of fellow employees and place those employees in danger. When these prejudices are refuted by work statistics, many employers simply fall back on the observation that seeing someone have a seizure at work frightens co-workers.

Absenteeism, injuries, and job performance are about the same for adults with epilepsy as for adults without epilepsy. There is a difference in some industries, such as manufacturing: people with epilepsy perform slightly *better* than people with no chronic health problems. Obviously, epilepsy does impose restrictions on certain types of employment. A person who has frequent grand mal seizures cannot safely operate a tractor, for example. The better-than-average safety on the job found in most studies of adults with epilepsy probably reflects the common sense exercised by these people. Thirty-seven percent of adults with seizure disorders claim that their choice of work was influenced by their disorder.

Hospitalization

When seizure control is very poor, hospitalization may be required to allow the physician to investigate the poor control and to make dramatic changes in antiepileptic medications. Unfortunately, frequent hospitalizations disrupt work, education, and family life; and yet hospitalization rates for all types of seizures have shown a general increase over recent years. As people with epilepsy get older, they are hospitalized more frequently for problems related to their seizure disorders, such as aspiration and injuries.

Women have been hospitalized at a consistently greater rate than men, by a factor of about 7 percent, over the past several years. This difference undoubtedly reflects a variety of social factors, since the types of epilepsy and the severity of problems faced by the two sexes are not significantly different. These social factors may include the more limited repercussions of hospitalizing a person who does not work outside the home, as opposed to taking a person away from a job, in the case of one-income families. Another social factor could be the uncertainty some husbands may feel in dealing with intractable seizures at home, as compared with the competence wives may feel. Or the different rates of hospitalization may simply mean that men are somewhat more assertive about getting professional care for their spouses than are women, or that they are more resistant to hospitalization for themselves. With changing patterns of employment and decision making in the family, this disparity between male and female hospitalizations may soon disappear.

Hospitalization should be considered only after a strenuous effort to control seizures in a normal environment has failed. The decreased stress, increased structure, and limited activity that are routine in hospitals may reduce seizures without any alterations in antiepileptic medication. But the benefits of this artificial environment disappear as soon as the person is discharged. The goal for patients is seizure control in the person's usual environment. This may require altering that environment, such as eliminating flash photography from the vicinity of a person whose seizures are triggered by flashing lights, or simply adjusting medication until the person can tolerate the everyday stresses of home and work without having seizures (Table 12).

Accusations of Malingering

As with any chronic disease, the person suffering from epilepsy has the option of exploiting it. Relatively minor problems with seizure control may be elaborated to gain sympathy, power, or freedom from responsibilities. In reality, exploitation of this neurologic disorder is unusual in adults, though it is often suspected by family members who cannot

TABLE 12

Circumstances That Can Lower the Seizure Threshold

Common	Occasional	Rare
Sleep deprivation	Barbiturate withdrawal	Specific noises
Alcohol withdrawal	Hyperventilation	Reading
Dehydration	Flashing lights	Sexual activity
Malnutrition		Eating
Infection		
Trauma		

believe that a long-term problem could be out of the victim's control.

Sometimes people with epilepsy are obliged to convince their families or co-workers that they truly do have a serious condition. Seizure disorders are so different from other chronic illnesses that people and their families often suspect they signal emotional disturbance rather than a neurologic impairment. Even when the family accepts the disorder as neurologic, the person with epilepsy may feel obliged to convince them repeatedly of its severity. Resentment often develops within the family if the person with the chronic problem is perceived as an opportunist.

A rift developed between a totally disabled young man, Eli, and his sister when he became eligible for social security because of his poorly controlled seizures. Although Eli had severe brain damage, his sister—who had been a good friend until the onset of the seizures—did not believe that he was actually disabled. She accused him of getting a "free ride" because he was "lucky."

Carter, who was forced to retire after he developed seizures from head injuries suffered in an automobile accident, faced repeated insinuations from friends and family that he was trying to build a strong case for litigation. His insistence that he was the victim of an accident was invariably greeted by skeptical remarks, and Carter became obsessed with proving that he was not perpetrating a fraud.

Much of the reluctance to recognize a family member's disability derives from an unwillingness to admit that a real tragedy has occurred in the family. The current cliché for this situation is to say that such a family is "in denial." Suggestions that the epilepsy is a "clever" or "useful" way to get out of work or to get disability benefits understandably offend the person with seizures, even though such remarks may just reflect the anxiety of friends and family who do not want to believe that the person with epilepsy is truly and irrevocably impaired.

Explaining Altered Behavior

When a generalized tonic-clonic convulsion occurs, there is little to explain to even the most uninformed observers. The victim loses consciousness, may suffer an injury, and is obviously confused after the most dramatic part of the incident. Less obvious seizure phenomena, such as bedwetting, staring spells, disorientation, nonsensical remarks, and disturbed speech, are more difficult for the person with epilepsy to explain. If he or she is determined to conceal the seizure disorder, then explaining this aberrant behavior becomes even more difficult.

Altered consciousness at an inopportune time can be devastating. Catherine, a 50-year-old woman with recurrent complex partial and focal motor seizures from a brain tumor, did not wish to reveal her medical condition by wearing identification. When the police found her confused and uncooperative in the midst of a traffic jam, they assumed she was drunk and placed her under arrest. Too confused by her seizure to follow their instructions to leave the car, Catherine was handcuffed, forcibly removed, and booked for resisting arrest. She was injured in the struggle and lost several thousand dollars' worth of cash and checks that she was carrying to the bank. Even though a physician wrote a letter explaining her behavior, she was obliged to appear in court to answer the charges brought against her.

Martin, who had both epilepsy and kidney disease, faced a similar predicament when police found him in a postictal stupor. They mistook his multiple dialysis punctures for track marks from drug abuse and arrested him as a presumed drug addict. His indignation when he recovered from his seizure did little to convince the police that he was anything but an offensive addict. Pleas that his doctor, rather than his lawyer, be called finally gained him credibility.

Sometimes people with epilepsy find themselves having to prove that an unfortunate incident was *not* caused by a seizure. Louise, a 24-year-old woman with fully controlled generalized seizures, had her driver's license revoked after an accident. She was struck by a car that went through a red light, and witnesses were willing to attest to where the fault lay. But the Bureau of Motor Vehicles demanded that she prove she was *not* having a seizure when the accident occurred. They asked for objective tests, such as an electroencephalogram, to document that she was seizure-free. Though no one at the scene held her responsible for the accident, the bureaucracy treated this incident as an accident involving a person with epilepsy, rather than as just an accident. Since no physician was in the car with her at the time of the accident, no one could provide an authoritative statement that she had not been having a convulsion. An abnormal electroencephalogram would not have meant she had poor seizure control, since people with epilepsy very often have abnormal EEGs between seizures, even on a dose of medication that controls seizures completely. In any case, the possibility of a normal EEG was eliminated by the extensive head injury Louise suffered during the accident. To make matters worse, the driver of the car that had run the red light, on learning that the Bureau of Motor Vehicles had suspended Louise's license, filed suit against her on the grounds that by driving with a seizure disorder she had recklessly endangered him.

These are admittedly gross examples of legal problems faced by people who develop altered behavior during a seizure, but they are certainly not rare. Much of the difficulty can be avoided if the affected person carries information about the seizure disorder in a conspicuous place, such as on a bracelet or necklace. A card listing seizure type and medications and carried along with identification provides more privacy but is more easily overlooked by nonmedical personnel.

Coincidental Problems

For many people, seizures are merely one facet of a disease of the nervous system that produces several disabilities. Over 75 percent of people with seizure disorders show some cognitive, behavioral, or other neurologic problem, such as weakness in a limb or vision impairment. In people with cerebral palsy, mental retardation and clumsiness may appear in addition to seizures; and in people who have suffered a stroke, paralysis and speech disorders may complicate the picture. In fact, seizures may be a relatively minor feature of the underlying disease with which a person must cope. The accident victim with paralysis of his right side, for example, may find his seizures to be little more than an annoyance in comparison with his other disability.

All of the individual's medical problems must be considered in managing epilepsy. A person may be uncooperative with doctors and nurses who are trying to suppress his seizures if he considers the seizures a minor problem in comparison with others that are being ignored.

Paralysis

Transient weakness in a limb or in an entire side of the body— a phenomenon called postictal or Todd's paralysis—occasionally develops after a seizure. The weakness rarely lasts more than a few minutes, but in some cases it lasts as long as 24 hours. Even brief weakness can be disabling if the person's work demands a constant level of physical performance, as in the case of a machine operator.

Regardless of its duration, postictal paralysis is not very common. Much more common is the association of seizures with paralysis that develops after structural damage to the brain from trauma, stroke, or tumor. When a person has had epilepsy for several years and then develops weakness or clumsiness on one side, an unsuspected tumor or vascular malformation in the head is probably responsible for both problems.

Dementia

About 15 percent of all people with seizure disorders are cognitively impaired. The impairment, which varies from slight memory disturbance to profound mental retardation, may be the person's principal difficulty. Although the vast majority of people with a seizure disorder are not mentally retarded, at least 60 percent of people who are mentally retarded have some type of seizure disorder. Many of the common misconceptions about epilepsy probably arose because people failed to make this distinction. Epilepsy does not cause dementia (that is, impaired thinking or memory), but some conditions that cause dementia also cause epilepsy.

Several types of seizure disorders are associated with memory problems. People with complex partial seizures frequently complain that they are not remembering new information as well as they did in the past. Ralph, a 52-year-old security officer who developed complex partial seizures in middle age, repeatedly hid bank books and other valuables and then forgot where he had put them. He also had trouble calculating change and keeping track of cash. Because the epilepsy had already substantially restricted his activities, his wife, Sarah, was reluctant to take his financial responsibilities away from him. All that was achieved by this consideration was increasing financial hardship for the entire family and growing anger at Ralph's incompetence. Rather than allowing resources to be lost because of her husband's memory disorder, Sarah eventually resolved the situation by taking all financial matters out of Ralph's hands. She decided that her husband's anger would cost her less than his dementia.

Prognosis

Both the adult with epilepsy and family members affected by the disorder worry about the long-term outlook. Insurance companies tell them that epilepsy increases the risk of early death, and friends tell of other people who were seizure-free after a few months of special diets, chiropracty, acupuncture, or other alternative health fads. The outlook, in fact, closely depends on the specific type of seizure disorder a person has and other health problems that are associated with it. Generalizations are difficult to make and unreliable for long-term planning.

Remission

Remission is the disappearance of all seizures in a person with a history of epilepsy who is no longer on any antiepileptic medication. Seizures that develop during adulthood or persist into adult life from childhood do not usually remit. This is especially true for people with abnormal electrical activity arising in the anterior temporal lobes. Not only will complex partial seizures associated with these temporal lobe disorders require medication for decades, but even with medication the seizures are often poorly controlled. Adults with any type of epilepsy are usually obliged to take antiepileptic drugs for the rest of their lives. Why seizures sometimes remit in children as they mature, but not in adults as they age, is unknown.

Adults who have remained seizure-free on antiepileptics for

several years are often eager to stop taking the drugs—to be rid of the expense, inconvenience, side effects, and the daily reminder that they are not "normal." It is not easy to tell how long an interval free of seizures is adequate before a person can safely attempt to give up medication. Some people free of seizures for four years will remain asymptomatic for life, and others free of seizures for ten years will have a convulsion within a week of stopping the medication.

Whether the EEG is useful in deciding when or if medication should be stopped is controversial. Brain wave abnormalities are not considered a good reason for continuing antiepileptic medications in a child who has been seizure-free for several years. In adults, the relationship between the brain wave patterns and the likelihood of recurrent seizures after years without seizures is very hotly debated. Most physicians agree that if no structural defect is evident in the brain and the EEG is normal after several years free of seizures, withdrawal of the antiepileptic medication can be attempted cautiously. This attempt should be made, of course, only if it is what the person wants. A person with a history of epilepsy must be aware that the seizures may recur when the medication is stopped.

Discontinuing antiepileptic drugs in the face of a persistently abnormal EEG is ill-advised. Stopping the medication at the start of a pregnancy endangers both the mother and the fetus (see Chapter 5).

Mortality

Premature death caused by a seizure disorder is a common fear. Although mortality statistics lend some support to this worry, the premature deaths that do occur among people with epilepsy are generally not caused by the seizures themselves. The ratio of deaths among people with epilepsy to deaths among people without epilepsy is 2.3 to 1; that is, a person with epilepsy is more than twice as likely to die at any given age as an identical person without epilepsy. But this mortality rate includes people who have seizures because of incurable brain tumors, massive head trauma, or fatal strokes. It also includes children who succumb to congenital neurologic damage, accidental head trauma, or infantile brain tumors that caused their seizure disorder.

In fact, if all people with ascertainable causes of epilepsy are excluded from the mortality statistics, the mortality for the remainder—that is, for people with idiopathic epilepsy—is close to that of the general population. There is little increased mortality in people with idiopathic generalized absence seizures or complex partial seizures, especially if seizures first appeared in adolescence and the person is female. There is no increased risk of early death in people with benign Rolandic epilepsy of childhood. As would be expected in any condition that increases the risk of accidental injury, increases in mortality rates are related to the severity of the seizure disorder (Table 13).

Mortality risk fluctuates over the course of the disorder. During the first two years after a person's first seizure, even if it is the only seizure ever observed, mortality is more than twice the expected rate. This increased mortality is largely a product of lethal conditions that caused the seizures in the first place, such as head trauma, stroke, or tumor. People with only one seizure who survive these first two years have normal mortality rates thereafter.

Mortality also shows a sharp increase for the interval 20–29 years after the initial diagnosis of the seizure disorder, a phenomenon that remains unexplained by current views of epilepsy and antiepileptic treatment. Also unexplained is the appreciably lower long-term mortality rate for women. Thirty years after developing epilepsy, the mortality ratio for women with epilepsy and women without epilepsy is 1.6 to 1. For men, that ratio is 2.1 to 1.

Certain types of seizures do have a poor prognosis. Myoclonic epilepsies, in which seizures with prominent mus-

TABLE 13

Factors That Lower the Risk of Death
among People with Epilepsy

Seizures are idiopathic in origin
Seizures are petit mal or complex partial type
Seizures are from benign epilepsy of childhood
Seizure control is good
Person with epilepsy is female
Seizures start in adolescence

cle jerks occur, increase the mortality rate more than fourfold during the first year after the appearance of the seizures. Myoclonic seizures are relatively uncommon, and many of the conditions responsible for these types of seizure disorders are lethal metabolic diseases. People who develop generalized tonic-clonic (grand mal) seizures are 3.5 times more likely to die during the first year than people in the general population. But again, it is symptomatic, not idiopathic, epilepsy, that drives up the mortality rates in both of these conditions. Generalized tonic-clonic seizures, for example, may be caused by viral encephalitis, which can be fatal.

Except for obvious intracranial causes of seizures and early death, such as meningitis, brain tumors, and strokes, no natural causes of death are notably prevalent in people with epilepsy. Accidents during seizures are responsible for some deaths in this group, but the most common causes of death in people with epilepsy are the same things that cause death in the general population—accidents, heart disease, and cancer. Status epilepticus, in which the person has repeated seizures without returning to normal consciousness, can be lethal if medical attention and effective antiepileptic treatment are not obtained soon after the appearance of the intractable seizures, although, again, death may be due to the underlying condition.

Accidents cause 5 to 16 percent of deaths in people with epilepsy, but whether a seizure caused the accident can rarely be ascertained. It is also inaccurate to blame antiepileptic drugs for the higher-than-expected incidence of accidents; excessive doses of such drugs may mildly impair coordination and slow response times, but in the most frequently lethal accidents, such as drownings, these factors do not play a major role. Some small studies suggested that antiepileptic drugs *decrease* mortality by protecting against heart disease, but long-term mortality figures have not borne out this early impression.

One cause of death that is inordinately common for people with seizure disorders is suicide (see Chapter 9).

Adjustment to Seizures

Adults with epilepsy and their families often face social and medical problems because of the neurologic disorder, but these problems are surmountable if they are approached with flexibility and patience. In most cases, the person who has frequent seizures will encounter the most difficulty adjusting to his disorder, maintaining a normal family life, and holding a job. But even adults with infrequent or easily controlled seizures may be deeply affected by the need to deal with epilepsy as a daily concern. Most people with seizures can achieve a productive and satisfying life, but achieving it may take considerable cooperation from family and friends. Common emotional reactions to the disorder, such as feelings of guilt and embarrassment, may incline the adult with epilepsy to withdraw from friends and relatives. Such withdrawal should not be allowed to end friendships and family ties.

Epilepsy usually can be adequately controlled so that it intrudes rarely, if ever, into the affected person's daily routine. Family and friends should treat it as an occasional inconvenience rather than as a perpetual tragedy. The adult with epilepsy never profits from being regarded as a functional cripple. Any family that treats the person with seizures as totally dependent should examine its motives for doing so. Even those people who face major restrictions on their activities because of the seizures or other nervous system problems associated with the seizures generally can and should develop lifestyles that maximize their independence and self-esteem.

Becoming and staying employed often play a major role in adjustment to the disorder. The people with epilepsy who are allowed to become totally inactive and dependent have the worst prognosis for sustaining a meaningful life. If familiar patterns of work become impractical because of the epilepsy, the affected person must be willing to make job or career changes. People who are forced by their illness to give up old employment goals must be encouraged to find new jobs that fit their changed abilities. Sometimes this means having to recognize and set aside delusions about miraculously returning to their old jobs. If a person has neurologic problems in addition to seizures, these must be addressed with rehabilitation or medication.

Medication, rehabilitation, and suitable work are pivotal in the social adjustment of most adults with epilepsy. The alternatives—inactivity and dependence—can demoralize the person with epilepsy and the family members on whom he or she depends.

Chapter Three

Marital Problems

If a person with epilepsy is married, many of the problems caused by the seizure disorder will affect the other partner in the marriage. The problems that develop may be economic and social as well as medical. Until a few decades ago, the appearance of epilepsy in a man threatened the economic survival of his family. With an increasing number of women working outside the home, a husband's seizures do not carry such grave economic consequences, but now a seizure disorder in the wife may drastically change the couple's standard of living. When both partners contribute to the family income, a work disability in either will affect the living standard of both.

Of course, the spouse of any person with epilepsy may lose a reliable partner in ways that go beyond economics. Childrearing, housekeeping, socializing, entertaining, sexual initiative, and other elements of the marriage must be redistributed, especially when the person's seizures are poorly controlled. If seizures are well controlled, the epilepsy may have little impact on either partner. But this often is not the case.

The spouse without epilepsy becomes responsible for sustaining the family in many respects. This extra responsibility may evolve into overresponsibility. A reasonable level of supervision of the partner with epilepsy may progress to obsessive surveillance. In trying to look out for the best interests of the person with epilepsy, a spouse may reduce the partner's life to a long list of prohibitions. Violation of the prohibitions angers the spouse who enforces them, and enforcement irritates the spouse who is subject to them. Resentment in both partners is often the outcome.

Increased stress in the marriage can result from sexual problems that may develop in people with seizures (see Chapter 4). The partner without epilepsy may turn elsewhere for sexual intimacy. Even if the marriage does not end, it may deteriorate into much less than a partnership. The epilepsy may be blamed for any friction that develops between spouses and may be used as a justification for excluding the affected spouse from decisions and activities that appropriately involve both partners in a marriage.

Frequency of Marriage

In the general population, about 69 percent of all men and 70 percent of all women marry. Among people with epilepsy, 56 percent of men and 69 percent of women marry. While marriage patterns for women with epilepsy are comparable to those of other women, for men they are not—a disparity that perhaps reflects a significant difference in social attitudes toward men and women with disabilities. Men with seizures are considered less reliable providers than men without seizures. Until very recently a woman's ability to provide financial support played a small role in the choice of a wife by most American men; in contrast, a man's potential as a provider was an important consideration when women chose a husband.

The age at which the seizure disorder first appears influences the likelihood of marriage. If the first seizure occurs after age 20, the affected person is as likely to be married or to get married as any member of the general population. Unfortunately, by age 20, 75 percent of the people who will develop epilepsy during their lifetime have already had their first seizure. The age at which complete seizure control is achieved also has an effect on marriage. For people whose epilepsy is fully controlled by the time they are 12 years old, marriage is as likely as for the general population. Men with epilepsy who marry even though they have had poorly controlled seizures since childhood usually separate or divorce in the first few years of married life.

Social factors probably influence these rates of marriage. Men have traditionally taken a more active role than women in proposing marriage. The basic element reducing marriage rates in men with epilepsy, especially epilepsy that begins at an early age, is probably a lack of assertiveness in seeking marriage partners, rather than the unwillingness of people in the general population to marry men with epilepsy.

Deception

Many people believe that revealing their epilepsy will destroy their chances of marrying. But when a person conceals epilepsy from a spouse until months or even years after they are married, the additional feeling of deception adds to the instability of the marriage. Deception is self-defeating, because it leaves the person with seizures feeling that the marriage can founder on one careless incident or remark, and it denies the partner without seizures the opportunity to decide whether to accept responsibilities that are not a part of the usual marriage contract.

When to discuss epilepsy is a dilemma for most people as they become emotionally or sexually involved with someone. It is awkward and usually considered socially inappropriate to discuss medical problems with casual acquaintances, but many intimate relationships start with casual acquaintance. If a long-term intimate relationship is likely, the epilepsy should be disclosed before dramatic changes in living arrangements are made. But it should be discussed in the same terms that any chronic medical problem, such as diabetes or arthritis, would be discussed.

If the person with epilepsy is uncomfortable with or uncertain of the facts, a doctor or another informed and articulate health professional should be asked to help in the discussion. Rather than simply announcing "I have epilepsy" and waiting for a terrified reaction, the person with epilepsy might say that a chronic problem involving the nervous system has been under treatment for some time and then explain, or allow a physician to explain, exactly what the problem is. A concerned lover should not be intimidated by a problem that is already being managed. Taking the initiative in disclosing the disorder allows the person with epilepsy to develop a frank and relaxed intimacy.

Common Fears of Spouses

To bystanders, generalized convulsions appear to be life-threatening. Even if the partner without epilepsy has seen grand mal seizures before and knows that death during a seizure is unlikely, other fears linger. Robert, whose wife had experienced more than one seizure a week for several years, commented, "I always try to wake her up when she has a seizure. I'm always afraid she'll go into a coma." Even when seizures are well-controlled, spouses worry constantly that the partner with epilepsy will have a seizure while driving or while walking near subway tracks or other dangerous locations. Family members often voice concerns about lethal accidents that can occur during seizures. Death, rather than additional disability, is the central fear.

Predictably, this fear is not often openly discussed by the two concerned parties. A middle-aged wife who was very outspoken in family group meetings about the dangers surrounding her husband because of his epilepsy admitted, "In my house, we don't discuss it." The rationale for this seems to be that imagining the dangers is upsetting enough; articulating them would only compound the fear. Unfortunately, maintaining this silence usually proves to be a substantial burden for the spouse who does not have epilepsy. One of the major values of family group meetings, in which several families with epileptic members get together to talk about problems at home, is that they give the whole family a safe forum for discussing such feelings. The opportunity to explore the fears often defuses them

Overresponsibility

Constant surveillance can become an obsession for the spouse of the person with epilepsy. "It's what we call the watchdog effect," explained Timothy, whose epilepsy had developed after brain surgery to remove a blood clot. "I sing in the shower loud enough so that Irene won't worry." The constant watching and worrying are a strain on both partners. One husband admitted, "I try to think of other questions to ask her besides, 'Are you all right?' I can never relax." In discussing the possibility of her husband's being arrested because of his confusion and erratic behavior, Phyllis remarked, "If you get arrested, I'll let them keep you. I need a day off."

With many types of seizure disorders, such as complex partial seizures, simply remembering to take medication can become a substantial chore. A man with poorly controlled seizures and frequent bouts of transient amnesia needed his wife, Wendy, to call his workplace every day to remind him to take his drugs on schedule. Even with this assistance, Jake would sometimes take out his pills, pour a glass of water, drink the water, and forget to take the pills.

Jake's disorientation and amnesia could last for minutes or hours. Wendy was understandably concerned whenever he deviated from his usual schedule; as she put it, "Even the dog got upset when he was late." Just as understandably, Jake felt entitled to alter his routine occasionally simply to provide himself with a little diversion. If Wendy tried to find him when he made an unplanned stop on his way home, he became furious. Her anxiety deprived him of independence.

Being the caretaker in this arrangement carries little reward. Even helping the person with epilepsy maximize the coveted independence goes unacknowledged. Techniques developed to help with drug scheduling or safety measures are often credited to the epileptic person's own ingenuity, even when it is the spouse who provides the technique. Credit is not given where it is due because the debt is too pervasive to acknowledge. As one weary wife explained, "I always have to be there to catch him, and I get angry, and I think, 'Let him fall.' I tell him to go lie down and he doesn't, and then he has a seizure, and I get angry, because he could have been upstairs in bed." Over and over her husband would try to assert control over the problem, rather than merely taking precautions, and each time that he failed she would have to deal with the consequences.

The spouse's tendency to take on excessive responsibility is especially annoying because it is a tangible reminder of the seizure disorder. Frank, a successful executive with seizures, commented, "If I hear her say, 'Are you all right?' one more time, I'll scream. It's a constant reminder that I'm not well anymore." Unfortunately, the watchdog relationship focuses so much attention on the person with epilepsy that the needs of other family members, including those of the ever-vigilant spouse, may be neglected. Frank felt extremely guilty when his wife became ill. But he only noticed that something was wrong with her when she stopped being so watchful of him. The person with epilepsy may resent the constant scrutiny and yet also fear that it will not be there. One young woman with seizures who was constantly trying to elude her husband's surveillance admitted that if he stopped being oppressively watchful she would assume her husband had given up on her.

Much of the overresponsibility is a reaction to poorly controlled seizures. As with other problems, overresponsibility usually fades as an issue when the epilepsy is fully controlled. When seizure control cannot be achieved, talking with others about one's frustration and resentment can help alleviate those feelings. Once again, the people best equipped to give advice on how to manage when seizure control is poor are other families faced with this problem. Contact with people in similar situations provides perspective, if not solutions. An issue, like the need to sing in the shower, that seems oppressive when the couple are alone at home quite often seems trivial when it is discussed in a family group meeting.

Loss of a Reliable Partner

The transformation that occurs with a seizure is transient, but the helplessness and haggardness that often appear with the seizure can be devastating to the spouse of the person with epilepsy. The husband of a young woman who developed frequent complex partial seizures abandoned all hope of having a real marriage. He had little physical contact with his wife and depended upon his mother in law to take care of her. A middle-aged woman whose husband developed epilepsy after more than twenty years of marriage described the day he had his first generalized convulsion: "When they took him out, they had an old man strapped in a chair. He was good for nothing. The doctors told me he was in limbo." Uncertainty over what the epileptic spouse will be able to do soon gives way to uncertainty over when the helplessness will recur. With antiepileptic treatment, many patients return to fully normal activities, but usually their spouses are left with the persistent image of someone active and able suddenly becoming dependent.

When seizure control is difficult to achieve, the disorder itself and the antiepileptic medication may combine to produce an inactive, sedated person. Tom had held two jobs for more than twenty years and had constantly painted and cleaned the house. After developing seizures in his fifties, he abruptly stopped working around the house. Frequent and protracted bouts of confusion forced him to retire from his jobs. His seizure control was poor despite antiepileptic medication, and he sat home every day staring out the window and watching television. "He's getting into not doing all the things he used to do," his wife, Laura, complained. "I know I have to give him more time, but he sits and does nothing. I can't take it. If you're going to die, die moving. Before the seizures, everything was automatically done. Before, I depended on him to do everything; now I do everything." Inactivity and loss of motivation are usually viewed as "giving up."

The spouse without epilepsy feels obliged to push the partner with epilepsy into activity, an obligation that leads to resentment. Mitchell, the husband of a young woman with post-traumatic seizures, was annoyed by his wife's sudden loss of energy: "I say fight back. It's too bad they're sick, but you can't let them go to sleep." Paradoxically, the spouse who pushes the partner with epilepsy into a more active life often resists the partner's initiatives to do things that might raise the risk of a seizure or accident. Laura, who had complained that her husband was no longer working around the house, was horrified one day to find Tom climbing a ladder outside the house to paint windows. Similarly, Mitchell spent uneasy hours every time his wife went off to the mall to shop. Even though both of these activities were familiar, they now posed unacceptable risks as far as the spouses were concerned. When Tom decided to fix a clogged gutter by climbing out onto the roof of the house, Laura became furious. She felt that so dangerous an activity was simply an expression of her husband's lack of "consideration." Risking injury was equated with denying responsibility for the family.

Laura may have been right to be upset. Refusal to avoid excessive risks *is* sometimes irresponsible, if not intentionally self-destructive. Linda, a nightclub performer who had experienced grand mal seizures since childhood, was seizure-free when she took antiepileptics regularly and got plenty of sleep, but she rarely did either. Whenever she felt well, she skipped medications, dabbled in illicit drugs, drank heavily, and partied late into the night. Such binges predictably provoked seizures, but neither Linda's boyfriend nor her parents could dissuade her. Their efforts to restrict her lifestyle only prompted more damaging behavior. She refused to be "limited" by her epilepsy.

Overprotecting the person who has epilepsy may go well beyond reducing the risk of accidental injury. An abiding fear that domestic problems will bring on a seizure may lead the family to shelter the person with epilepsy from day-to-day stress. Problems with the children or with finances are hidden. Excitement over parking tickets, unpaid bills, and school problems are all avoided. In many cases, the epileptic spouse feels bitter about being excluded from crises. One middle-aged man with complex partial seizures complained, "You're not even called upon to do what you're expected to do as a parent and a husband. It's the same as saying, 'You're not capable and so we're not calling you.'" A young woman explained, "It's like being thrown in a closet."

The costs of maintaining a stable environment around the person with epilepsy include resentment in the protective partner and anger in the partner whose disability is emphasized by the protection offered. While the partner with epilepsy may vent his feelings freely, the spouse without epilepsy cannot voice her resentment because of fear that the complaint will upset the delicate balance that spares the family the burden of recurrent seizures. The often outspoken complaints from the spouse with epilepsy about exclusion from family responsibilities may compound the protective spouse's feelings of being misunderstood and unappreciated.

Isolation

Social isolation afflicts the spouse without seizures as much as it does the person with epilepsy. The husband of a woman with unexplained seizures complained, "You find people are afraid of you. It's like you have something more than epilepsy, like the plague." Misconceptions and prejudices that seemed rather innocuous in family members and friends before the epilepsy developed become a source of constant annoyance and interference. Neighbors may stop visiting, out of concern that their children will be upset or even emotionally injured by seeing a seizure. Myra and Ron, a couple with young children, were unable to get a 14-year-old neighbor to babysit because of the concern of the girl's parents that Ron would be erratic or violent or simply sick while the babysitter was there. This aversion to sickness is not unusual and not confined to epilepsy, but it is erroneous to believe that a person with epilepsy is likely to have a frightening or dangerous episode at any moment.

Social isolation extends even to near relatives. Like friends, family members may fear that a seizure will occur while they are around. Sheila, a young woman whose husband, Will, developed epilepsy within a few weeks of their marriage, found her mother's reaction at first confusing and then annoying. The mother had done volunteer work in hospitals and had never shunned the company of sick people. But when Sheila revealed that Will had epilepsy, her mother stopped visiting their home and became remarkably unhelpful. When the couple had a child, the new grandmother refused to be in the house with the baby and Will unless Sheila was also there. Sheila's mother claimed that her main fear was that her son-in-law would hurt himself, but why this prevented her from spending more time with her daughter and grandson was never discussed.

Sheila's mother proved disruptive when a seizure actually did occur. Instead of trying to help, she screamed and cried. In her panic she left Sheila alone to deal with the seizure and forced the couple's child to leave the room. The young boy, Patrick, who had often seen his father have seizures and helped out by placing cushions around him, was more frightened by his grandmother's reaction to the seizure than by the seizure itself. In discussions with Sheila, her mother insisted that Will was taking too much medication for his own good, but also that more must be done to eliminate his seizures.

Other members of the family were no more helpful than the mother-in-law. Visiting the homes of brothers and sisters became difficult for the couple because the family would not adjust to Will's needs. Even though his seizures were predictably triggered by flashing lights or watching television, when he visited Sheila's family they all continued to watch video games and television. At extended-family activities, photographs were taken using flash attachments. Will was effectively excluded from most family activities simply because his relatives refused to alter their patterns of entertainment even slightly when he tried to participate.

Neighbors and friends may also be unhelpful or disruptive by offering useless advice. "They make you feel like you're doing something wrong," one woman explained. "They ask if you've ever tried some medication they see mentioned on television." Much of the information provided through such channels is absurd, inaccurate, or simply banal, and explaining to a well-meaning friend or relative why the advice should not be followed can be a substantial chore. When a couple dismisses the advice as useless, friends or relatives often become offended. They do not realize how tiresome it becomes having to deflect so many intrusive suggestions.

Even medically sophisticated people can be a burden. Christopher was questioned by a nurse, who elaborated on all the dangers his wife, Melissa, faced because of her seizure disorder. The young man commented, "I want to leave when people start telling me what I should do. I'd like to say, 'Mind your own business. You couldn't possibly know what we know about it now.'" Doctors unfamiliar with Melissa's case would tell Christopher that he must be mistaken about details that he had repeated during more than a dozen hospital admissions. His long and close association with Melissa's illness made him much more sophisticated about the problem than the majority of the medical personnel he had to deal with, and perceiving this made him feel even more isolated.

Most families with epileptic members do not realize that many other people face this same predicament. Once the feeling that this family problem is unique is dispelled, much of the fear and hopelessness can be eliminated. Discussions with others in similar dilemmas can relieve the tension that inevitably develops in unhelpful exchanges with relatives, friends, and health care providers.

Struggles with Autonomy

People with epilepsy often complain that their spouses are too intrusive, too watchful, or too involved in their lives, but the spouses complain that the partner with seizures is constantly trying to exclude them from a problem that affects them both. Camille, the wife of a dialysis patient with poorly controlled partial and generalized seizures, complained that her husband was most unwilling to discuss his seizures when they were at their worst. "Sometimes I try to talk to him," she explained, "but he says it's nothing." It seems that people with epilepsy do not want anybody to notice their seizures—even their husbands and wives. "He does not believe that he disturbs us," suggested Mary, the middle-aged wife of a man with complex partial seizures. "He thinks there is something wrong with me . . . not him." Even though the seizures were extremely disruptive in the lives of both partners, Mary's husband resisted involving her in managing them.

One man who developed seizures after an automobile accident justified this desire to exclude his wife by claiming that her attention was condescending and even dictatorial. Michael explained, "I sense that she's always on the edge of her chair. She's always watching me." Some people with epilepsy feel that involving their spouses in controlling the seizures deprives them of the little self-control and responsibility they still have. Discussing these kinds of friction with other couples who know from their own experience what the problems are makes the issues between the spouses much less abrasive.

Infidelity and Divorce

The constant strain of dealing with epilepsy makes divorce a very real consideration. "At what point will I break?" asked the husband of a young woman who developed seizures within weeks of their marriage. "I've never been married to a normal woman." He could not help wondering what a relationship with a woman unburdened with this problem would be like. The wife of a middle-aged man with complex partial seizures admitted, "I'm always screaming, 'Divorce!' . . . The worst part of it is when you go through a period of getting better." After hope develops that daily life can be fairly normal, the return of seizures is especially devastating.

The sexual problems that accompany poorly controlled epilepsy may deprive the nonepileptic spouse of a sexual partner and lead to infidelity. How often infidelity is a consequence of sexual deprivation under these circumstances is unknown (see Chapter 4). Often, issues around intimacy and infidelity can be used as an excuse to end an exhausting and unsatisfying relationship. If the spouse without epilepsy turns to a sexual partner outside the marriage, the spouse with epilepsy can feel simply wronged, rather than deserted, and the spouse without epilepsy can claim provocation for the infidelity. Infidelity is a more socially acceptable reason for divorce than an inability or unwillingness to cope with epilepsy.

Defusing Marital Problems

There is obviously no single approach to help ensure the stability of an intimate relationship. When a marriage shows signs of falling apart because of the strain of epilepsy, family counseling is appropriate. Group meetings of families with epileptic members can also be useful in this context. Insights into how to deal with specific marital problems emerge when a group of couples share their own techniques and failures.

When Margarita first joined such a group, she expected her marriage to end within a year; she felt she had to leave her husband because he was incapable of coming to terms with his seizure disorder. After several months of meeting with other women in similar situations, Margarita recognized that *she* could not accept his disorder, and this insight, curiously, defused the problem for her. She had felt that she was a failure as a wife; but after talking to other equally frustrated wives, she realized that it was the neurological problem, not their shortcomings as spouses, that was eroding all their marriages.

Epilepsy puts strains on marriages and other intimate relationships, but it need not be the reason for ending these relationships. Both partners must recognize what problems are being fostered by the seizure disorder and then look for techniques to minimize them. The partner without epilepsy often does not realize how much of his or her anger and resentment derives from feeling overresponsible for the person with epilepsy. Allowing the epileptic partner to take charge of whatever he or she can reasonably do will reduce much of the friction in these relationships. The partners with epilepsy, in return, must learn not to expose themselves or their families to excessive risks.

When seizure control is poor, sexual issues often arise that aggravate problems already facing the couple. Additional stress may come from friction with other family members, who react to the epilepsy with fear or disbelief. All of these difficulties usually can be surmounted if the couple is willing to discuss them. Such discussions may not work well if they are limited to the affected couple, because neither partner can be objective. What usually does help is going to a family counselor or sex therapist, who can identify the difficulties and guide the couple in resolving them.

Chapter Four

Sexual Activity

People with epilepsy face the same sexual problems and exhibit the same abnormalities found in the general population, but with a slightly higher frequency. In some cases the sexual dysfunction may be directly related to the epilepsy or its treatment, and in other cases the connection is debatable. Whatever their origin, sexual problems are as treatable in people with seizures as they are in everyone else. Anticipating difficulties that may develop and addressing them aggressively will spare epileptic individuals and their partners much frustration.

Risk of Sexual Dysfunction

Almost any group whose sexual behavior is subjected to long-term medical observation will appear to have more sexual problems than "normal" people. People with epilepsy fall into this category and seem to have a slightly elevated rate of sexual dysfunction. In reality, they may have little, if any, more sexual difficulty than the general population; the more detailed information available about them may just highlight their problems. Furthermore, as the sexual practices of the general population come under closer scrutiny, the definition of "normal" sexual activity is becoming more and more inclusive. In the future, investigators may conclude that sexual dysfunction among people with epilepsy falls well within the normal range.

With these qualifications in mind, one can fairly say that most people with epilepsy lead normal sex lives. But for certain people (such as those with complex partial seizures) and under certain circumstances (such as poor seizure control) sexual function may be adversely affected. In most instances, the main problem is a lack of interest rather than an actual inability to perform or engage in sexual activities. Fear that sexual intercourse or excitement will cause seizures may inhibit not only the person with epilepsy but the partner as well. Other kinds of sexual dysfunction are rare in people with epilepsy, although sexual eccentricities such as transvestitism and fetishism do occur in some people with complex partial epilepsy (see Table 14).

Controlling seizures will not eliminate all of these sexual problems. In fact, efforts to treat seizures can cause problems of their own. Some people lose their sex drive (libido) as a side effect of antiepileptic medications. Others may develop distressing cosmetic problems with long-term use of antiepileptic drugs, and these changes in appearance may undermine the patient's self-confidence in pursuing sexual intimacy.

Among established couples, sexual inhibitions and anxieties develop primarily when seizure control is poor. The simplest, but often the most elusive, solution to this problem is improved seizure control. When that is not feasible, other ways must be found to minimize the disruptive effects of the disorder. Substantial barriers to the resolution of sexual problems are the reluctance of many patients to discuss their sexual difficulties and the reticence of many physicians in asking

TABLE 14

Sexual Dysfunctions Described
in People with Epilepsy

| Hyposexuality |
| Transvestitism |
| Fetishism |
| Exhibitionism |
| Drug-related impotence |

detailed questions about sexual behavior. When the problem
has been fully identified, it is more easily remedied.

Sexual Problems with Complex Partial Seizures

Decreased sexual activity (that is, hyposexuality) is common
in both men and women with this type of seizure disorder. It is
not simply a reaction to chronic illness: hyposexuality occurs
in 50 percent of people with complex partial seizures but in
only 30 percent of people with other chronic medical disorders, including grand mal seizures. Hyposexuality is not properly a sexual "complaint," since most people with complex
partial seizures do not complain about their lack of interest in
sex. If any complaints are offered, they usually come from the
sexual partner of the person with epilepsy.

Impaired Libido
Lack of sexual interest, rather than inability to perform, is primarily responsible for low rates of sexual activity among people with this disorder. Affected men are not physiologically
impotent, and affected women do not have pain with intercourse; they simply lack interest in initiating sexual activity or
in responding to the initiative of others. Many people whose
complex partial seizures started before puberty or at puberty

remain without sexual experience throughout their lives. If complex partial seizures start later in life, after a sexual relationship has become established, the patient's partner will usually notice a profound deterioration in sexual interest.

Most people do not realize that this seizure disorder itself can affect libido, by interfering with normal hormone secretion. The patient often believes the antiepileptic medication is responsible for a loss of sexual interest, while the patient's partner may suspect that the patient is still sexually active but with another person. Both of these conjectures are dangerous. The patient is tempted to stop the antiepileptic medication in an attempt to restore sexual appetite, and the neglected partner not only starts to doubt the affected person's honesty but feels wronged and abandoned.

The best that can be offered to the frustrated and anxious spouse is a frank assessment of the situation. The sexual interest of the partner with complex partial seizures is not likely to return to its former level, though good seizure control sometimes helps. The spouse must decide whether the relationship is satisfying enough in other ways to justify its continuation despite sexual frustration. And of course some partners may welcome a lessening of libido in their spouses, if it corresponds with their own waning interest in sexual activity.

Sexual Eccentricities

People with complex partial seizures have more than the expected incidence of sexual behavior that people in the general population consider to be eccentric, aberrant, or even deviant. This includes exhibitionism, fetishism, and transvestitism. Exhibitionism is a desire to be seen by another person in sexually provocative poses, such as unclothed or engaged in intercourse. Fetishism is attachment to and arousal by items, such as shoes or underwear, that are not always considered sexually charged. Transvestitism is an obsession with wearing clothes usually worn by the opposite sex.

If the seizures begin in adulthood, the eccentric sexual behavior may appear after years of more conventional sexual interests. The basis for this change in sexual preference is unknown. Sexual eccentricities are not part of the seizure itself: the patient has no disturbance of memory or alteration of consciousness when performing the sexual activity. The behavior usually occurs during the interictal period, the time when the patient is not having any obvious seizure activity.

A few people, most of whom are women, do exhibit atypical sexual behavior during the aura of the seizure, during the seizure proper (the ictus), or during the postictal confused phase. Stereotyped activities (automatisms) that may occur include undressing, masturbating, or, rarely, attempting to stimulate other people. Behavior during these periods of altered consciousness may be in stark contrast to the affected individual's usual sexual behavior. One woman who was frigid between seizures would become highly receptive to sex during her seizures. Men with this type of seizure disorder often have protracted erections (priapism), but they do not commit sexual attacks or other clearly purposeful sexual advances. Rape is not a feature of sexual seizures.

Orgasm with Seizures

A very few patients with complex partial seizures—again, almost all of them women—have orgasm as part of their seizures. In most of these women the orgasmic seizures occur premenstrually, and sexual satisfaction persists long after the seizure is over. When the orgasm occurs during the aura, the patient is able to recall enjoying it. Some patients are tempted to allow their seizure control to deteriorate in order to have these orgasmic seizures.

Some women report pleasurable sensations in the groin during the aura, and these are accompanied by vaginal secretions characteristic of sexual excitation, but no orgasm follows. Sexual seizures have never been observed in prepubertal girls, and the few men who report changes in genital sensation with their seizures have unerotic or unpleasant sensations. In women, the seizures seem to originate in the right temporal lobe. This is consistent with reports from neurosurgeons who perform surgery to manage poorly controlled seizures: stimulation deep in the temporal lobe during the operation occasionally elicits erotic feelings in these women patients.

This type of sexual arousal may be more common than is reported, since most people do not volunteer information about their sexual feelings. If it is more common, then it may have substantial effects on people with complex partial seizures. In any case, the fact that these orgasmic phenomena occur almost exclusively in women suggests that seizures involving the temporal lobe affect sexual function in men and women quite differently. Sexual appetite and activity may be increased in some women with temporal lobe seizures. Even if a woman's sexual behavior changes only during the seizure itself, her exhibitionism, genital manipulation, and sexual receptivity during that phase may have considerable impact on her sexual partner, for better or worse. Whether her partner is indifferent, excited, or dismayed by this sexual display will have consequences for their relationship.

We do not yet know if changes in sexual activity are transient phenomena or if they are permanent side effects of complex partial seizures. So-called deviant sexual behavior is observed more often in patients with temporal lobe epilepsy developing before age 3 than in the general population. All that can be concluded from this observation is that people with early temporal lobe epilepsy express different sexual preferences from their peers. It may be that they simply give less inhibited answers to questionnaires about sex. Even when a patient's behavior is atypical for the social setting, the behavior is not necessarily pathological. In some countries, a person appearing naked on a public beach or in a public park is considered an exhibitionist, whereas in other countries the same behavior is considered normal.

Other Causes of Poor Sexual Adjustment

A person with epilepsy may have sexual problems that are totally unrelated to the seizure disorder. If a patient has impaired sexual function without impaired interest, the seizure disorder is probably not responsible for the dysfunction. All men who are unable to achieve or maintain an erection (that is, who are impotent) and all women who experience pain during intercourse (a condition called dyspareunia) should be investigated for other possible causes of these disorders.

The type of sexual dysfunction should always be considered in the diagnosis. A man with complex partial seizures who has normal erections and ejaculations but feels no excitement at the time of orgasm is more likely to have a central nervous system problem associated with his epilepsy than a man who simply cannot have an erection. A woman who achieves no vaginal lubrication despite feeling considerable excitement at the time of intercourse should be investigated for a peripheral nerve or vaginal problem, even if she has poorly controlled seizures.

Occasionally, antiepileptic drugs are responsible for poor sexual performance, at least in men. Phenobarbital and primidone (which is partly converted to phenobarbital) sometimes cause impotence. When a patient's libido is intact and no evidence of peripheral nerve damage can be found to explain his impotence, a change in antiepileptic medication is appropriate. Replacing phenobarbital with phenytoin (Dilantin) or replacing primidone with carbamazepine (Tegretol) or one of the newer medications may completely eliminate the sexual dysfunction.

Fear of Seizures during Sex

Sexual activity rarely triggers seizures. Nevertheless, if a seizure does occur during sexual intercourse, it can be devastating for both partners. People with epilepsy generally avoid activities that they believe will lead to seizures, whether that belief is based on experience or superstition; the fear of having a seizure can lead a person with epilepsy to initiate sex less often and can interfere with sexual enjoyment while having sex. A seizure during lovemaking may be even more upsetting to the partner without epilepsy, and if a person first learns of a lover's seizure disorder in such a traumatic way, he or she may be an especially reluctant partner in the future.

Some people worry, during sexual intercourse, that the exertion of intercourse will cause their sexual partner or spouse to have a seizure, and this fear can interfere with the couple's ability to enjoy sex. One wife's extreme attention to her husband's expression and movements made him too self-conscious to become fully aroused and reach orgasm, despite sexual encounters that could last over an hour. The abnormal breathing pattern, the altered expression, and the stiffening of limbs that accompany normal sexual excitement in both men and women can resemble seizure phenomena, and this resemblance can make both partners too nervous to relax and allow excitement to lead to orgasm.

Overcoming this sexual inhibition is difficult even with the most uninhibited couples, but it is often impossible with couples who cannot talk frankly, or at least accurately, about their sexual problems and techniques. A counselor can assure the couple that a seizure during intercourse should not pose any special problems to either partner and that a seizure is no more dangerous during sex than at other times, but this reassurance may not dispel the worries of the partner without epilepsy. Both partners may find it embarrassing to tell other people, even medical personnel, that the patient lost consciousness and had a seizure during sexual intercourse. Reassurance that this is unlikely may do little to improve sexual performance or satisfaction.

Couples must be patient and committed if they are to overcome the sexual inhibitions that develop when epilepsy is poorly controlled. Where considerable sexual dissatisfaction has developed, the couple should explore the possibility that a mutual tendency to withdraw from each other as a reaction to the epilepsy is making their sexual troubles more intense. Here again a family therapist can often help. Where there is little more to the sexual problem than anxiety, counseling with a sex therapist is often helpful.

Cosmetic Effects of Antiepileptic Drugs
Contributing to the social and sexual problems of young people with epilepsy are the cosmetic changes that often accompany anticpileptic therapy. Severe acne can develop when bromide is used to treat seizures, but this drug is rarely prescribed now that other antiepileptics are on the market. But other commonly used drugs also cause skin changes. Phenytoin (Dilantin) and, to a lesser extent, phenobarbital can cause coarsening of facial skin and darkening of facial hair. Arm and leg hair may also darken and appear thicker, but this is much less of a problem than facial hair for young women.

Both men and women suffer from periodontal problems associated with phenytoin, particularly gingival hyperplasia (the overgrowth of the gums; see Figure 4). This condition can lead to loss of teeth unless patients submit to repeated gum surgery. Careful attention to dental hygiene reduces this risk. Some women on valproate (Depakote) notice a tendency to gain weight and lose hair. A variety of rashes can occur with several antiepileptic drugs; these often signify allergic reactions that may call for a change in medications.

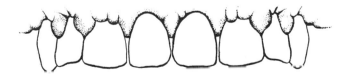

FIGURE 4.   Gingival hyperplasia. In this condition, the gingiva extends over the teeth and produces a space between the teeth and gums in which debris can accumulate. Periodontal disease will develop unless repeated gingivectomies are performed.

Effective treatment of these cosmetic problems is essential, at least in children and adolescents, because unless these side effects are controlled, patients may refuse to take their medications. Many people would rather risk occasional seizures than have unattractive gums and lose their teeth. Switching to another drug may avoid further problems with skin, hair, and gums, but the existing changes will not disappear without some type of intervention. If scalp hair remains thin after medications are changed, minoxidil (Rogaine), which stimulates hair growth, can be tried. Gingival hyperplasia can be resolved with gum surgery (gingivectomy) and rigorous dental care. Hair on arms and legs may require shaving or chemical removal. These approaches also work for facial hair, and some women find them acceptable. For other women, electrolysis is a better approach, since it is more permanent, is less likely to produce stubble, and does not carry the masculine associations that face-shaving does.

Remedies

Most people with epilepsy can and do have normal sex lives. Specific problems can develop with some types of seizures and certain antiepileptic drugs, but most of these are surmountable. Some patients with longstanding complex partial seizures have little interest in sex, but even this symptom often abates with changes in seizure control or antiepileptic medication. Whenever sexual dysfunction develops, the couple should recognize that the epilepsy or its treatment may be causing it. If the partners begin exchanging accusations or assume that the problem is untreatable before they seek remedies, both will suffer from the loss of the relationship.

Sexual dysfunctions are usually not caused by permanent changes in the epileptic partner. Sexual activity can usually be restored to the way it was before the epilepsy if the sexual partners can frankly discuss their problems. A sex therapist or physician should be involved in the investigation and treatment. In many cases all that is needed to correct the problem is a change of antiepileptic medication, discontinuation or a change of drugs used for conditions other than seizures, or professional counseling to minimize the sexual inhibitions and fears the partners may have developed in response to the epilepsy.

Chapter Five

Childbearing and Inheritance

Separate from the sexual and marital problems associated with epilepsy are the concerns that develop when a couple thinks about having children. The decision about whether to have children is often affected by the frequency and severity of the seizures experienced by the spouse with epilepsy. The couple often wonder if their offspring will inherit a seizure disorder and if the parent with epilepsy will be able to care for the child. If it is the wife who has epilepsy, concern about birth defects from antiepileptic medications may dominate the couple's worries.

Reproductive Rates

Over the past forty years, epilepsy has become less important in determining whether a person has children, but it still plays a significant role. Certain problems more common in people with epilepsy than in the general population, such as severe mental retardation and other major handicaps, prevent some

TABLE 15

Marriage and Reproduction

Men with epilepsy:
Marry less often than women with epilepsy
Have less sexual interest than other men

Women with epilepsy:
Have fewer children than men with epilepsy
Have fewer pregnancies than other women

In both men and women with epilepsy:
Marriage rates are normal if seizures are
controlled by age 12
Marriage rates are lower if uncontrolled
seizures begin before adolescence
Families are smaller than in the general
population

people with seizures from having children. But even those without these obvious limitations have fewer children than do people in the general population (see Table 15). Reproductive rates are depressed for both men and women with epilepsy. Women with epilepsy who marry have only 69 percent as many live-born children as do married women in the general population. Men with epilepsy who marry have as many children as the average married man, but fewer men with seizures marry.

Many factors influence this lower rate of reproduction. The specific type of seizure disorder seems to affect the reproductive rate. Complex partial seizures, for example, are often associated with a decrease in sexual interest. A woman with seizures who lacks sexual interest might marry for reasons other than sexual attraction, but she would probably have fewer pregnancies than women without epilepsy because she would avoid sexual intercourse. Overall, including those who never marry, women with complex partial seizures have an average of 1.6 children each, compared with women in the general population, who have 2.1 children each. Men with this type of seizure disorder have an average of 0.5 children each, as compared with 2.1 among men in the general population. These differences probably reflect differences in the rates of marriage for women and men with complex partial seizures.

Any statistics on reproduction must be interpreted with caution, because people do not always answer questions on such a sensitive topic honestly, even when anonymous questionnaires are used. A woman whose husband is uninterested in sex or fatherhood may still have children, either by never using contraception and hoping that rare sexual encounters with her husband will result in pregnancy or by finding another sexual partner. If a man with an affected wife has a child with another woman, this child will not count in surveys of children produced by his marriage.

Married women with epilepsy seem to have fewer children than other married women simply because they do not become pregnant as often. Their rates of miscarriage are no higher than those in the general population (14 percent), and the seizure disorder itself does not seem to affect ovulatory cycles or cause hormonal problems that decrease fertility. Antiepileptics have no apparent effects on the unfertilized eggs in a woman's ovaries, and the number of eggs released by women with epilepsy, whether on antiepileptic drugs or not, appears to be the same as that for women who do not have epilepsy.

Some women make a conscious decision not to reproduce. Jessica, a woman in her late twenties whose complex partial seizures had been poorly controlled for several years, told her new physician that both she and her husband had decided against having children for professional reasons. But after switching to a new regimen of antiepileptic drugs and being seizure-free for four months, Jessica and her husband began asking about the dangers her drugs would pose to a fetus if she became pregnant. With the threat of seizures abating, the couple's views on having a family changed.

When seizures are well controlled, a parent with epilepsy can provide as much support, direction, and instruction for children as a parent without epilepsy. But the possibility that the disorder will cause problems in the future even though it is now under control inhibits some couples from becoming parents. The physician most familiar with the patient's seizure disorder should be able to estimate the future burdens likely to be imposed by the epilepsy. A parent with poorly controlled seizures cannot be relied upon to take full responsibility for a newborn infant, but the same person may be an excellent parent for a 4-year-old. A parent with frequent seizures should not be left to bathe a newborn alone but can play with and teach the older child. Obviously, the resources and support available to each couple and the roles each spouse is willing to play should be fully and objectively assessed when deciding whether or not to have children.

Eleanor, a recently married 28-year-old woman with generalized tonic-clonic seizures, insisted that her career goals compelled her to avoid having children, but she contradicted herself when further questioned about her impressions of motherhood. She explained that her seizure disorder—which had recurred after years free of sciznres—was of unknown cause and might be hereditary. She said her parents "had a nightmare with the epilepsy when I was a child. If it weren't for all the illness, they could have enjoyed themselves and had some money now." Though her father insisted that they had not suffered because of her epilepsy, Eleanor went on to discuss the special risks her child would face because she would have to take antiepileptic drugs throughout the pregnancy. Despite her avowed lack of interest in childbearing, she had accumulated a great deal of information on the birth defects associated with her antiepileptic regimen.

A person who wants to have a child but whose partner is unwilling has several options. If the marriage is of value to both spouses, professional counseling from either a marriage counselor or a sex therapist might be profitable. Artificial insemination from a donor may be an option for a woman whose husband is impotent. When the wife has epilepsy and is worried about the dangers of pregnancy more than about raising a child, an impartial assessment by a physician of the risks involved for both the mother and the child may be helpful.

Potential parents who hesitate out of concern about inheritance of epilepsy should consult the physician most familiar with the patient's problem. The physician can give the couple a realistic estimate of the chances that a child will be affected or can refer them to a genetic counselor for an assessment of the risks. Adoption may be a possibility for couples who conclude that the risk of inheriting epilepsy is too high to have biological children.

Pregnancy

Women with epilepsy usually have uncomplicated pregnancies, normal deliveries, and healthy children. But it is also true that pregnancy presents special problems for the woman with epilepsy (Table 16). Epilepsy can affect a woman's pregnancy, and the pregnancy can affect her epilepsy. A woman who is on an antiepileptic drug must deal with changes in the way the medication is metabolized during the pregnancy, as well as with the effects the medication could have on the fetus. If she is on no medication, pregnancy may increase her seizure rate. Even women who have never had seizures before may develop them during pregnancy and require medication. In that situation the question arises whether to continue antiepileptic medication after the pregnancy has ended.

Effects of Pregnancy on Medication

Most antiepileptic drugs are metabolized more rapidly during pregnancy. This means that drug levels in the blood will fall as the pregnancy progresses and make the woman more vulnera-

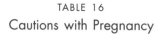

TABLE 16
Cautions with Pregnancy

Metabolism of antiepileptic drug changes
Seizure threshold changes
Anesthetic technique must be adjusted
Newborn may be sedated
Antiepileptic drug may be in breastmilk

ble to seizures unless the dosage is increased. The rate at which the antiepileptic drug level falls is unpredictable. Measuring the level every few weeks during the pregnancy is the best way to assess changes. An effective level can be maintained by simply increasing the dosage, but subtle factors, such as the binding of the drug to proteins in the blood, complicate the interpretation of drug levels.

The additional dose required generally increases during the second and third trimesters of pregnancy, but the decision to change the dose of medication should be made in close consultation with the woman's neurologist, who is familiar with the behavior of the drug and the pregnant woman's medical history. Increasing the amount of medication usually will not increase the side effects. Most side effects depend on what gets into the blood, not what goes into the stomach.

Any risk that medication may cause defects in the developing fetus is greatest during the first trimester of pregnancy, so there is no reason to allow the mother's level of antiepileptic protection to fall during the second and third trimesters. Immediately after the end of the pregnancy, the dose of antiepileptic drug required will decrease. To avoid an overdose at this point, the medication must be reduced, again with the rate of change dictated by changes in the level of antiepileptic medication in the blood. Within a few months of delivery or termination of the pregnancy, the woman will usually require the same dose of antiepileptic medications to control her seizures as she needed before she became pregnant.

Effects of Seizures on the Fetus

Good control of seizures is as important for the developing fetus as for the pregnant woman. Some women stop taking their antiepileptic medication in anticipation of becoming pregnant or as soon as they realize they are pregnant. This places the fetus at risk of injury from seizures. Although the developing embryo will not develop seizures of its own simply because its mother is having seizures, it will have to deal with the profound chemical (metabolic) changes that accompany some seizures. Generalized tonic-clonic (grand mal) seizures often start with abnormal or interrupted breathing. This causes a dramatic drop in the level of oxygen in the blood and a sharp rise in carbon dioxide levels and blood acidity. These changes, which may last minutes or hours, create an abnormal environment that may be harmful to the fetus. Additional damage to the fetus may occur if the woman injures herself during the seizure, a not uncommon occurrence with both generalized and partial seizures.

Effects of Pregnancy on Epilepsy

Epilepsy commonly surfaces in vulnerable people who are under extraordinary stress. Pregnancy may not be an extraordinary physical stress for most women, but it does involve hormonal changes, and these hormonal changes may trigger a seizure disorder. When the seizures occur without other apparent changes, they may be the first indication that the woman has epilepsy. When seizures occur in association with high blood pressure and changes in kidney function, the woman is said to have eclampsia or toxemia of pregnancy. Seizures that first occur during labor are more worrisome than those occurring earlier in the pregnancy, because they may be caused by bleeding from defects in the blood vessels of the mother's brain brought on by the exertion and agitation of labor, or from some other serious neurologic condition, such as a brain tumor, that had not previously caused symptoms.

For a woman with longstanding epilepsy, the exhaustion, pain, and lack of sleep associated with protracted labor may be stressful enough to induce a seizure. For a woman with a low seizure threshold, minimizing the length of labor and the intensity of the pain is an important consideration during labor, but this does not mean that a cesarean section is preferred for women with epilepsy. The reasons to have a C-section are the same for women with epilepsy as for other women. A C-section is more physically stressful than an uncomplicated vaginal delivery after a short period of labor. The simplest and least stressful approach to the delivery can be decided only by the expectant mother and her obstetrician. Despite the best-laid plans, what happens during labor will affect the decision.

A seizure at any time during or shortly after pregnancy may be no more than the recurrence of a longstanding but unrecognized problem. Young women who develop seizures while pregnant may have no memory of seizures they suffered in infancy. Because of the variety of possible causes of seizures during pregnancy, treatment is not a simple matter.

Seizures caused by a correctable metabolic problem, such as a low level of calcium or sodium, may be fully controlled without the use of antiepileptic drugs. If an obvious metabolic problem is found, it should be corrected before antiepileptic drugs are considered. Any seizure not caused by an obvious metabolic problem should be treated with antiepileptic medication until the cause of the seizure can be established. Even if it occurs during the first trimester—the period during which fetal development is most likely to be affected by antiepileptic medications—and even if only one seizure has occurred and its cause is not apparent, antiepileptic medications should be prescribed. Seizures during pregnancy can never be viewed as benign incidents. They must be investigated and treated, regardless of when they occur in the pregnancy, but in both investigation and treatment the risks to the fetus must be considered.

Both the mother and the physician should be reluctant to conduct extensive investigations during a pregnancy; those requiring radiation, such as a computed tomogram of the brain (CT scan), or other tests that might damage the fetus should be delayed unless an induced abortion is planned. A spinal tap, in contrast, will not disturb the pregnancy and will reveal if bleeding has occurred into the spinal fluid. Ultrasound studies of the brain also pose no risk to the fetus and may provide evidence of abscesses, blood clots, or other large masses inside the head. A more thorough neurologic investigation with radiographic studies is appropriate after the pregnancy has ended. A woman who develops seizures during pregnancy may have a vascular malformation or a tumor that was not obvious until the stress of the pregnancy made the problem symptomatic.

Treatment of Seizures during Pregnancy

What medication should be used to suppress idiopathic seizures that first occur during pregnancy depends upon the type of seizure and the stage of pregnancy. If seizures appear during the first three months of pregnancy, the antiepileptic drugs most likely to cause birth defects should be avoided. This means that phenytoin, primidone, and phenobarbital are inadvisable early in the pregnancy unless the woman was on these medications before she became pregnant. Whether phenytoin poses more of a risk to the developing fetus than primidone or phenobarbital is controversial. Any of these drugs should be avoided if possible. Other drugs occasionally used as antiepileptics, such as acetazolamide (Diamox), which do not consistently suppress seizures during pregnancy should also be avoided. Trimethadione is an antiepileptic generally not used by American physicians because of problems with toxicity, such as fetal malformations.

Which medication is best for a particular woman depends on many factors, and both a neurologist and an obstetrician should be involved in the final decision. For many women, especially with complex partial seizures, carbamazepine is the drug of choice. Despite concern that valproate (Depakote) might cause disturbed neural tube closure and produce spina bifida, a disturbance of spine formation, this drug has been relatively benign when taken by most pregnant women.

Changes in the medication regimen early in a pregnancy have their own dangers and are not advisable. In many cases, the mother has been on an antiepileptic, such as phenytoin, for several months before she realizes that she is pregnant. Changing the drug from one that has been well-tolerated by the mother to one for which there is no experience in that patient is a risky business. The risks to the fetus and the risks to the mother should be candidly discussed by the physician before any alterations in treatment are attempted.

Seizures during Labor

If seizures first occur during labor, an oral antiepileptic may be impractical and intravenous medication may pose unnecessary complications for the anesthesiologist. Intramuscular phenobarbital or fosphenytoin (Cerebyx) may protect the patient from further seizures during the delivery without producing significant sedation of the mother or the newborn, though any antiepileptic given near the time of delivery must be considered a potential problem for the newborn as well as for the mother. If the dose of phenobarbital is high, the physician must be prepared to deal with a sedated infant.

However, allowing the mother to face recurrent seizures during labor in order to spare the child exposure to antiepileptics is even riskier to the infant, as well as to the mother. Both mother and newborn are better off if the mother is given enough antiepileptic medication to stop the seizures, even if that means intravenous doses of fosphenytoin, phenytoin (Dilantin), diazepam (Valium), lorazepam (Ativan), or phenobarbital. But the physicians involved must pay close attention to blood pressure and breathing patterns in both the mother and the newborn.

Birth Defects

Most children of women with epilepsy have no birth defects. For women with epilepsy who do not take antiepileptics and do not have seizures during pregnancy, the incidence of birth defects is only slightly increased above that of the general population. The reason it is increased at all is probably that some idiopathic seizure disorders are part of hereditary syndromes that can produce birth defects as well as seizures. If the woman with epilepsy is on a single antiepileptic drug, the risk of having a child with a birth defect increases to two to three times that faced by the general population, but it is still small.

The most common birth defects caused by antiepileptic drugs are cleft lip or palate, heart malformations, and hip dislocations. Cleft lip is twelve times as common as in the general population; heart anomalies are eighteen times as common; and the relatively rare problem of congenital hip dislocation is forty times as common. But it must be emphasized that even a forty-fold increase in a very rare occurrence is still very rare.

Women who required antiepileptic drugs before pregnancy must be assumed to require some medication during pregnancy to avoid damage to the fetus from seizures. Still, a concerted effort should be made to keep the pregnant woman's drug intake to a minimum. Breaking down the dose into multiple doses over the course of the day can help to even out the level of the drug in the blood and minimize peak levels. The highest rate of birth defects (almost 13 percent) occurs in women who are taking more than one antiepileptic drug and yet have seizures during pregnancy. Even when only one drug is used, the risk of birth defects varies with the drug taken. An important exception to the general rule to minimize drug exposure during pregnancy is the need to supplement phenytoin (Dilantin), carbamazepine, valproate, and perhaps other antiepileptic drugs with the vitamin folate to minimize the risk of neural tube defects.

All of the well-established and widely used antiepileptic drugs—phenytoin (Dilantin), carbamazepine (Tegretol), primidone (Mysoline), valproate (Depakote), phenobarbital, and acetazolamide (Diamox)—appear to disturb fetal development to a lesser or greater extent, especially during the first trimester, but which will have the most impact on a particular person is largely unpredictable. Serious malformations of the face, heart, or skeleton appear in about 10 percent of infants whose mothers take phenytoin during the first trimester, and the majority of these babies show slow growth and development for the first few months or years. There is no way to predict how severely a given fetus will be affected by exposure to phenytoin; even twins may be affected differently. If phenytoin is given during the first trimester, it must be supplemented with the vitamin folate.

Some studies have implicated carbamazepine (Tegretol) and valproate (Depakote) in spina bifida (failure of the neural tube to close). People with a family history of any type of failed neural tube closure, such as spina bifida, encephalocoele, myelocoele, or myelomeningocoele, should avoid these two drugs. The more recently introduced antiepileptics—gabapentin (Neurontin), lamotrigine (Lamictal), felbamate (Felbatol), topiramate (Topamax), tiagabine (Gabatril), and vigabatrin (see Chapter 11)—have uncertain or unknown effects on the fetus, but it is generally assumed that they all carry risks.

Diazepam (Valium) is not effective as an antiepileptic when taken orally, but it is effective against generalized seizures when given intravenously. Many women, whether they have epilepsy or not, take diazepam during pregnancy to deal with anxiety. The effects of this medication on the fetus are controversial, but current evidence suggests that it does not cause birth defects.

The most serious fetal defects can usually be detected in the first or second trimester, through alpha-fetoprotein screening (which uses a blood test), ultrasound (which uses sound waves), or amniocentesis (a procedure in which amniotic fluid is extracted from the uterus and subjected to genetic analysis); if a severe defect is detected, abortion is an option for some women. Unfortunately, many women do not plan pregnancies, and even when the pregnancy is considered probable it goes unrecognized until the end of the first trimester. It is during this three-month interval that fetal development is most likely to be disturbed by exposure to antiepileptic drugs or a depressed serum folate level. Reducing antiepileptic levels at that point or trying to eliminate multiple drug use may do little to protect the fetus from drug effects and may substantially increase the risk to the fetus from seizures.

For all of these reasons, a woman with epilepsy who plans to keep any fetus that she conceives, whether intentionally or incidentally, should maintain an antiepileptic regimen during her fertile years that will be optimal for a fetus as well as for her. She and her partner should discuss the issue of fetal malformations and the risks of multiple drugs early and often with her physician.

Because of interference with vitamin K metabolism by some antiepileptics, women with epilepsy should receive 20 mg/day of vitamin K1 during the last few weeks of their pregnancies. This should help protect the fetus against bleeding. The newborn should receive 1 mg of vitamin K intramuscularly at birth.

We do not yet know what effect antiepileptic drug use by the father has on offspring. Most of the problems faced by the developing fetus are from exposure to antiepileptic medications while in the womb, but it is quite possible that sperm and eggs can be damaged before conception. If such damage occurs, it must be relatively rare for obvious defects to have eluded detection for so long.

Breastfeeding

Women who nurse their infants generally need not be concerned about the level of antiepileptic medication in breastmilk. Some antiepileptics, such as phenytoin, may be found in breastmilk in minute amounts, but they do not seem to cause problems for the developing infant. Phenobarbital may be transferred in sufficient quantities to sedate the newborn, but this does not appear to have long-term adverse consequences. For most of the newer antiepileptic medications, such as lamotrigine (Lamictal), gabapentin (Neurontin), tiagabine (Gabatril), and topiramate (Topamax), the significance of drug secreted into breastmilk is unknown. Of course, a woman should tell the physician prescribing any drug that she is breastfeeding.

The Inheritance of Epilepsy

Epilepsy usually appears in just one member of a family. The child of a man who develops epilepsy after a gunshot wound to the brain is at no greater risk of developing epilepsy than the child of a man shot through the lung is of developing shortness of breath. This is not to say that epilepsy never occurs in several members of a family. Some of the diseases that cause seizure disorders are inherited; this is why the likelihood of developing epilepsy increases if other members of a person's family have epilepsy that is not caused by an injury or an infection in the nervous system. But epilepsy itself is not properly considered a hereditary disease.

For both normal and abnormal genetic traits, the simplest patterns of inheritance are called dominant, recessive, and

X-linked. A dominant trait will appear if a person inherits the relevant gene from either parent. A recessive trait will appear only if a child receives two relevant genes, one from each parent. X-linked traits are inherited only in men, and only if they receive a defective X chromosome from their mother. This is because the X chromosome men receive from their mother is the only X chromosome they have (it is paired with a Y chromosome inherited from their father), whereas women have two X chromosomes (one from each parent) and no Y chromosome. When a man inherits an X chromosome that carries the defective gene, he will exhibit the X-linked trait. In women, on the other hand, the effects of an abnormal X chromosome from either parent are offset by the normal X chromosome from the other parent.

Inheritance is more complicated than this simplified version suggests. Even when an abnormal trait is dominant, the likelihood that it will appear varies, depending on its "penetrance." Thus a father with tuberous sclerosis, a disorder with many possible nervous system complications, may pass on the gene for the disorder to his child, and yet the child may exhibit a much milder version of the trait than the father does.

Hereditary problems that may cause epilepsy include defects in brain formation (including blood vessels in the head), disorders of metabolism, and recurrent tumors. Occasionally an adult without epilepsy will have a hereditary neurologic disorder that can cause epilepsy in his or her offspring. The inherited defect may be nothing more than an abnormality in electrical activity in the brain. Presumably such an abnormality results from a metabolic problem in the brain, but the chemical basis for it is not apparent with currently available tests.

The rate of epilepsy in the general population is 1 or 2 in 200. If we take all causes of epilepsy in adults into account (accidents as well as inherited disorders), the risk for a child with one epileptic parent is five times that of the general population. But that still places the risk at only 2 to 5 children out of 100. In the case of adults with seizure disorders that exhibit a dominant pattern of inheritance, the risk that a given child of the affected person will have the disorder may be as high as 50 percent. In the case of fraternal (nonidentical) twins, if one develops epilepsy, there is a 5 to 20 percent probability that the other twin will develop it. In the case of identical twins, if one twin develops epilepsy, the chance that the other one will too is 30 to 90 percent.

A child is at highest risk of developing epilepsy if the affected parent is the mother and if she has generalized (petit mal or grand mal) seizures of unknown cause and with no aura (see Table 17). Regardless of which parent has the seizure disorder and what type of seizure the parent has, sons are slightly more likely to develop epilepsy than daughters. For the offspring of a parent with any one of several types of epilepsy, the incidence of seizures runs as high as 12 percent, but this disturbingly high figure includes children who have only one seizure in childhood and never develop a persistent seizure disorder. Unequivocal epilepsy will develop in 2.9 percent of the sons of women with all types of epilepsy, 2.3 percent of the daughters of women with epilepsy, 1.1 percent of the sons of men with epilepsy, and 0.6 percent of the daughters of men with epilepsy. Although the differences between these rates are small, they are statistically significant.

Why children of an epileptic mother are more likely to develop the problem than children of an epileptic father is unknown. Part of the statistical difference may be caused by mistaken identity: the wrong man is much more likely to be identified as a parent than the wrong woman. Another explanation is that birth complications play a part in the development of some seizure disorders, and women with epilepsy are more likely to have complicated pregnancies and deliveries than women without epilepsy.

Children who develop hereditary seizures unrelated to a metabolic problem follow a fairly predictable pattern. The

TABLE 17

Factors Which Increase the Risk That a Child Will Inherit Epilepsy

The mother has seizures

The child is male

Either parent has idiopathic generalized seizures

Several family members have epilepsy

A metabolic disease associated with epilepsy occurs in relatives

seizures usually appear between the ages of 5 and 19 years. The type of seizure is generally the same as that observed in the parent, but the age of onset for the child may be slightly earlier than that reported for the parent. A noteworthy exception to both of these rules occurs if the parent has simple partial (focal) seizures. Children of parents with simple partial seizures often develop generalized tonic-clonic (grand mal) or generalized absence (petit mal) seizures, which usually surface by age 2 if they are going to develop at all.

Occasionally a child will be the first family member recognized to have epilepsy. Other relatives with "drop attacks," episodic confusion, blackouts, and temporary memory lapses will be diagnosed as suffering from epilepsy only after the child develops seizures. If a child has recurrent seizures, the likelihood that his parents have a tendency to have seizures may be as high as 14 percent; his siblings, 3 percent; his distant relatives, 2.8 percent.

In some families a specific disorder causing seizures is not inherited but a general susceptibility to seizures of one type or another is inherited. A hereditary lack of resistance to viral infections of the brain, for example, may increase the likelihood that certain nerve cells in the brain will be damaged. The brain injury could cause epilepsy, and the epilepsy would appear more frequently in members of this family, even though the family members share a problem with immunity rather than with the structure or function of the nervous system. This may explain the appearance of several different types of epilepsy in the same family. The most dramatic example of this is in the case of complex partial seizures. Although most of the known causes of these seizures are not hereditary, 2.6 percent of the relatives of people who suffer from them will have some form of epilepsy.

Commonly Inherited Types of Seizures

Some types of epilepsy exhibit well-defined hereditary patterns. The classic form of generalized absence (petit mal) attacks is one of the most common hereditary types. True absence attacks are transmitted in a dominant pattern, but people who carry the gene or genes responsible for this disorder do not necessarily have actual seizures. They may just exhibit the electroencephalographic pattern typical of people with generalized absence attacks. A child will usually develop actual petit mal or absence seizures between the ages of 5 and 9 if the attacks are ever going to occur. Of those children whose electroencephalograms show the typical pattern, 25 percent will develop seizures. Thirty-five percent of the offspring of people with this electroencephalographic pattern will show the same pattern, at least during childhood, even if seizures never develop.

Benign febrile seizures, which do occur more often in related people than in the general population, are not strictly speaking a form of epilepsy. Just as seizures will occur in some people who have low levels of calcium in their blood, seizures will occur in infants in some families when these children have high fevers. Benign febrile seizures invariably occur between 6 months and 5 years of age and only at the peak of a rapidly rising fever. The tendency to have these relatively benign and transient seizures appears to be transmitted in a dominant manner with variable penetrance.

A seizure disorder called Rolandic or benign focal epilepsy of childhood, which occurs in older children and resolves completely as the child matures, also seems to be dominantly inherited. Rolandic seizures are focal seizures, but generalized seizures may also occur, and whatever seizures develop are most often during sleep. These seizures are easily controlled with antiepileptic medications and stop by the end of adolescence.

Several different types of metabolic problems affecting the brain are inherited and cause epilepsy (see Chapter 10). In such cases the seizures may be the most obvious initial sign of the disease; this gives the false impression that the epilepsy, rather than the biochemical problem, is inherited. One such disorder is myoclonic photosensitive epilepsy, a dominantly inherited problem in which flashes of light precipitate seizures. The patient usually has a brief trance, often with small jerking movements of the limbs and trunk. On the electroencephalogram this may look very much like petit mal. Children may induce these seizures by waving their hands in front of their eyes or by watching a flickering television screen. This seizure disorder actually may be the initial sign of a metabolic disease, such as Lafora body disease, that causes central nervous system damage and produces a myoclonic epilepsy.

Hereditary Nervous System Diseases

Many hereditary diseases of the nervous system cause seizures as a symptom. The seizure disorder is rarely the only symptom of the hereditary disease, but it is quite often the initial or most prominent one.

Disorders Apparent in Infancy

Most of the metabolic problems that cause seizures during infancy also cause mental retardation. Although the chemical bases for several of these disorders have been identified, treatment is available for very few.

Phenylketonuria (PKU), one of the most common metabolic causes of seizures and mental retardation in infants, is also one of the most treatable. The blood of a newborn can be checked for abnormal handling of the amino acid phenylalanine. If the tests indicate PKU, a diet low in phenylalanine may prevent significant retardation and epilepsy. Even if a woman's phenylketonuria is well managed, so that she shows no sign of the disorder while on a careful diet, her children will be damaged by the disorder during pregnancy. The chemical abnormalities in the pregnant woman's blood, while presenting no significant problems for her, may have a devastating effect on her developing fetus. Children of women with PKU invariably have learning disabilities and seizures because of brain damage induced by the mother's abnormal blood composition. This means that women with phenylketonuria should be advised not to have children. The child of a woman with PKU is not likely to have PKU itself but is extremely likely to suffer severe nervous system damage.

Another inherited disorder that can cause seizures is Tay-Sachs disease, a problem common in some groups of Ashkenazi Jews. As much as 3 percent of this population carries genes that will lead to a deficiency in the enzyme hexosaminidase A. Children who inherit this gene from both parents will develop seizures, progressive eye damage, and severe mental retardation. Tay-Sachs is a lethal disorder, and its victims rarely survive past 3 years of age. It can be detected in the sixteenth week of pregnancy by amniocentesis, and earlier with chorionic villus sampling, a technique that takes cells from the placenta. Parents may choose to have an induced abortion before the defective fetus matures. Carriers of the gene can be identified before pregnancy through genetic testing.

Less common but equally lethal metabolic disorders include several defects in metabolism of fatty materials (lipids). In

Niemann-Pick, infantile Gaucher, and Krabbe disease, various materials accumulate abnormally in nerve cells and cause damage to the nervous system. All of these unusual metabolic disorders are recessively inherited.

Several dominantly inherited problems are relatively common and not invariably lethal. One of these is acute intermittent porphyria, an enzyme disorder that often interferes with normal brain function. This became infamous as the cause of recurrent insanity in many of the royal houses of Europe during the eighteenth century. King George III, the English monarch during the American Revolution, suffered from this metabolic disturbance.

Most of the X-linked diseases causing seizures are progressive disorders of the entire nervous system. Other symptoms are likely to overshadow the seizures, and the victims usually die in childhood. Treatment of seizures in these patients is frustrating because the progressive character of the diseases interferes with the development of an effective drug regimen.

Tuberous Sclerosis
Tuberous sclerosis is a hereditary disease that may cause little more than pale spots on the skin or may lead to profound mental retardation and seizures. It is a dominantly inherited disorder, and one child out of every 30,000 to 100,000 will develop the disease, but the severity of symptoms is remarkably variable and impossible to determine at birth. Common signs of this disease, other than seizures and mental retardation, include whitish spots on the skin, fibrous growths at the bases of the nails, and tumors in several different organs, including the brain, eye, kidney, and heart. Eighty-eight percent of people with the disease will have seizures, including all of those who also exhibit mental retardation. Sixty percent of the victims of tuberous sclerosis are retarded; and if seizures develop before a child is 2 years old, that child will be retarded.

Neurofibromatosis

Von Recklinghausen's neurofibromatosis, a hereditary disorder that affects the skeleton and skin as well as the nervous system, is dominantly inherited and appears in one out of 3,000 births. Twelve percent of the victims of this disease have seizure disorders, and many of these also have nervous system tumors, some of which are lethal. People with neurofibromatosis have lumps in the skin caused by benign tumors of the peripheral nerve-lining cells and hyperpigmented spots, called café-au-lait spots, that extend over several centimeters.

Although the condition is dominantly inherited, it has a variable penetrance. What type of seizures will develop is determined by what part of the brain develops abnormal structures or tumors. Many people with this disease remain free of seizures all their lives despite obvious tumors along nerves in the skin.

Huntington Disease

Huntington disease is a dominantly inherited disorder that usually causes abnormal movements and progressive mental deterioration. About 10 percent of patients with this disorder have seizures. A "rigid" form of Huntington disease, which usually develops in children or adolescents, has a much higher incidence of seizures. These children experience rigidity, tremor, and diffuse slowing of movements similar to those of an elderly person with Parkinson disease. About 85 percent of children with this rigid form will have epilepsy. This is a slowly progressive disorder for which no treatment is available.

Genetic Counseling

In a family with a clearly defined hereditary problem, it makes sense for couples to seek genetic counseling before they decide whether to have a child. In some populations, people who are told the risks of having a child with a hereditary disorder tend to have more children than similar people who are given no counseling. The parents of an affected child are inclined to suspect that any future child will be similarly affected. When they are told that the risk of having another child with the disorder is only one out of four or one out of two, they are more likely to have other children.

Even if their second child also has, say, tuberous sclerosis, they assume that the probability of having a normal child increases if they simply keep trying. In fact, the risk that any particular child will be affected is exactly the same as that for previous children. If the risk of inheriting a nervous system disorder is fifty-fifty for the first child, it will be fifty-fifty for the tenth child, even if his nine siblings all have the disease. Genetic counselors stress that inheritance is like coin-flipping: each flip of the coin is equally likely to turn up heads or tails, regardless of what turned up on previous tosses.

As more prenatal tests are developed to detect hereditary disorders that can cause epilepsy, more parents will be able to conceive, have the tests, and then decide whether to abort the fetus if it is abnormal. It would obviously be more desirable to avoid conceiving a defective fetus at all, but this type of genetic selection is still far from practical. Couples who are at high risk of having children with epilepsy should be given what information is available, including information on prenatal testing, and allowed to decide on a suitable course for themselves. If they decide to have no children or to adopt children, they should be directed to medical or social agencies that can help them realize these choices.

Chapter Six

The Child
with Epilepsy

Seizures are common in infancy, childhood, and adolescence. Some type of seizure occurs in as many as 8 out of every 1,000 children. Occasionally the seizures disappear as the child matures, but in most cases epilepsy that appears in childhood will persist into adult life. About 80 percent of all people who have epilepsy are children or else they developed the problem when they were children. The family problems and conflicts that will result from epilepsy in a child usually depend on the severity of the epilepsy. Well-controlled seizures may pose few real problems; poorly controlled seizures may become the focus of all family activities.

With poor seizure control, parents often feel obliged to restrict the child's life and sometimes their own lives as well. The child may be preoccupied with fears that the seizures will be lethal or crippling. Even when seizures are fully controlled, family interactions that developed as a response to the earlier poorly controlled seizures may continue long after their usefulness and appropriateness have ended. A mother's protectiveness may be necessary when close supervision is essential for seizure control, but if that protectiveness persists after the seizures cease to be a problem, or even after the child becomes an adult, it can undermine the relationship and make it difficult for the person with epilepsy to have a normal life.

Overprotectiveness sometimes forces a child with epilepsy into the role of being the permanently "sick" member of the family. The sick role evolves in reaction to the threat of illness as much as to the reality of a chronic problem. The relationships that develop among the "sick" child, the parents, and siblings may have disadvantages for each family member, but those relationships will still be difficult to alter and may persist indefinitely.

Families with children who have epilepsy face special challenges, but the outlook is far from bleak. New medications and techniques are introduced every year which improve seizure control and minimize the effects of the disorder on both the child and the family. Most children growing up with epilepsy can lead virtually normal lives, both inside and outside their families.

Causes of Seizures in Childhood

Children develop epilepsy for many of the same reasons as adults (see Chapter 10), but there are some noteworthy differences. Hereditary metabolic problems, with seizure disorders as an early symptom, are much more likely to appear in childhood than in adulthood (see Chapter 5), whereas brain tumors are more likely to cause seizures in adults than in children. Some infections and injuries that cause seizures are acquired before or during birth, though the seizure disorder that results can last a lifetime. Accidental poisoning, which can cause seizures, is a minor hazard for adults but a major threat to children. Head injuries cause brain damage and seizure disorders at all ages, but children face different risks from head injuries at different stages in development of the skull and brain. In short, children are not just small adults; and consequently the causes, complications, and treatment of seizure disorders in infants and children will not be the same as in adults.

Epilepsy in childhood may develop within hours of birth or late in adolescence. The age at which it appears is often related to the type of seizures or to their cause. Certain patterns of epilepsy, such as salaam attacks—brief episodes in which the child thrusts its arms forward as it drops its head—invariably appear in infancy. Other seizures, such as myoclonic fits—involving limb jerks that may knock the child to the ground without causing altered consciousness—are more typical of the first year of life and adolescence. If a metabolic problem is responsible for the seizures, the age at which seizures begin will depend on the pace at which the metabolic disease disrupts the normal interaction of brain cells. Epilepsy may appear within the first few months of life in infants with Tay-Sachs disease and not appear until adolescence in people with ceroid neuronal lipofuscinosis, even though both of these rare nervous system diseases involve the abnormal accumulation of materials in brain cells (see Chapter 5).

Disorders Present at Birth

Children are often born with a defect of the central nervous system that immediately or eventually causes seizures (see Table 18). It may be caused by an injury at birth, a hereditary metabolic problem, or a structural abnormality that developed during the pregnancy. When seizures developing in infancy or childhood can be traced to a discrete injury, the most common one is inadequate oxygen supply to the brain during or just before delivery. This condition, called birth asphyxia or birth anoxia, is often presumed to be the cause of seizures that develop in any child who had problems breathing at birth or who was delivered with the umbilical cord tightly bound around its neck. But this view is overly simplistic. The fetus

TABLE 18
Causes of Seizures in Newborns

Birth asphyxia

Intrauterine infection

Metabolic disorders

Head injury

Congenital brain malformation

Intracranial hemorrhage

Drug withdrawal in addicted mother

does not take its first breath until after it is outside the womb, and by that point the cord has been removed and cannot interfere with air flow. Theoretically a tight cord could interfere with blood flow to the brain before birth and thus reduce the oxygen supply to the fetus, but the cord would have to have a powerful grip on the neck, and that is improbable until the fetus is well advanced in the birth canal.

Problems with breathing at birth may in fact be a sign of injury to the brain rather than the cause of it. Inherited metabolic diseases do not wait until after birth to cause brain damage. And in the case of premature infants, fragile blood vessels in or near the brain may start to bleed during birth, causing brain damage. Intracranial bleeding during labor may be the unsuspected cause of both seizures and poor breathing in a premature newborn.

This does not mean that an inadequate oxygen supply to the brain during birth is not a major source of perinatal injury. Even when other causes of perinatal damage are taken into account, birth asphyxia is the most common cause of brain damage at birth. Failure to provide the brain with adequate oxygen irreversibly destroys nerve cells and causes other adverse changes in the brain. Epileptic activity develops from the increased irritability of the injured brain, and the extent of the damage determines what signs of nervous system injury besides the seizure disorder will appear as the child develops. Injuries caused by insufficient oxygen to the brain at birth are loosely grouped together under the term cerebral palsy. Epilepsy does not invariably develop with cerebral palsy, and when it does it may appear years after all other neurologic problems caused by the birth injury have stabilized.

In some instances, an infection acquired before or at birth causes brain damage that later produces seizures, along with slow cognitive development, limb weakness, poor coordination, or other neurologic disorders. A variety of intrauterine infections, including toxoplasmosis and cytomegalovirus (CMV), may cause fetal brain damage that results in seizures months or years later. Some infections are contracted during delivery. For example, exposure to the virus *Herpes simplex* in the birth canal may cause encephalitis (inflammation of the brain) that leaves the infant with a low seizure threshold. The risk of injury to the central nervous system is high enough that a cesarean section is often performed when this type of infection is present in the birth canal.

The entrenched view that forceps are a common cause of brain damage during birth is unsupported by objective evidence. Forceps, properly applied and handled, protect the fetal skull and speed the infant's transit through the birth canal.

When brain dysfunction is apparent within the first few weeks of life, the underlying disorder may be an inherited metabolic disease, rather than an inadequate oxygen supply during birth. If the metabolic disorder causes substantial damage to the gray matter of the brain, seizures often develop, sometimes even before birth. The chemical or hormonal disturbance in this type of disease may be at the cellular or glandular level. Tay-Sachs disease does its damage at the cellular level, through the failure of cells to eliminate metabolic waste products. Other metabolic dysfunction may result from an impaired thyroid, adrenal, pituitary, or other gland vital to normal growth and development.

Treatable metabolic disorders are exceedingly uncommon, but they are always worth looking for, just in case. One rare cause of seizures in newborns that can be treated is pyridoxine dependency. Infants with this disorder need high levels of pyridoxine, a B vitamin, in their diets to avoid mental retardation and seizures. More easily diagnosed metabolic problems include abnormal handling of calcium and magnesium. Newborns are routinely screened for chemical disorders of the blood, which are usually easily corrected.

In addition to hereditary errors of metabolism, seizures in childhood may also arise from developmental defects in the central nervous system. A child with a large portwine spot on the face, for example, may have Sturge-Weber syndrome, a developmental abnormality that causes vascular malformations in the brain and elsewhere, with associated brain damage and seizure disorders.

Head Injury

Brain damage from head injuries is very common in children (Table 19). Automobile accidents alone make head injuries a major public health problem, but added to this is the trauma sustained in falls, sporting injuries, and child abuse. In the most common form of head injury, the front of the head hits a hard object, with possible damage to the frontal and temporal lobes of the brain (Figure 5). These are the areas of the brain where seizures usually develop.

In young infants, the bones of the skull are not fused, and openings in the top of the skull (the fontanelles) are large enough to allow direct injury to the brain. The custom in some cultures of molding the head by binding it tightly after birth can cause trauma to the infant's poorly protected brain, but most children survive this deformation without injury. Binding inflexible materials, such as wooden boards, over the

TABLE 19
Causes of Epilepsy in Children

"Cerebral palsy"

Head injury

Congenital malformations

Poisoning

Metabolic disorders

Nervous system infections

Brain tumors

Vascular malformations

fontanelles can cause brain damage that may not be manifest until years later, when seizures appear. Brain injury can also occur without any apparent skull fractures. In such cases, discharge of blood mixed with spinal fluid from the nose or ears of an infant may provide more unequivocal evidence of injury than a skull x-ray.

Child abuse can produce many long-term adverse effects, one of which is seizures. That a child does not develop epilepsy within hours or days of a beating does not mean the condition will not subsequently develop. Children at special risk are those who lose consciousness or have evidence of skull fractures and intracranial blood clots.

In children as in adults, generalized tonic-clonic (grand mal) and complex partial (psychomotor) seizures are the most common types of seizure activity that develop after head injuries. In most cases the character of the injury determines the type of seizure, but in some cases a family history of seizures may lead to epilepsy after relatively minor head trauma. By contrast, children who are at no special risk of developing seizures may suffer major head trauma without ever having seizures. This simply means that a predisposition to develop epilepsy may be as important in some post-traumatic seizures as is the head injury itself.

Febrile Seizures

Sometimes children with high fevers develop seizures, usually generalized convulsions entailing a loss of consciousness. Between birth and age 5, about 2 percent of all infants have febrile seizures and 1 percent have seizures unrelated to fevers. If the seizure occurs between 1 year and 5 years of age, is associated with a fever, is nonfocal, lasts less than 15 minutes, and is not associated with a metabolic disorder or central nervous

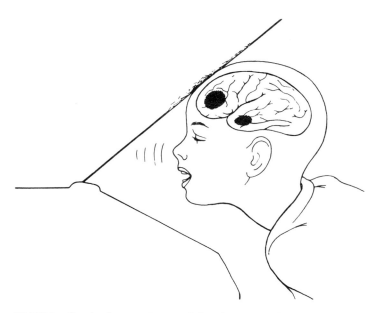

FIGURE 5.   Cerebral contusions with head trauma. If a person's head strikes a windshield during an automobile accident, injury to the brain may occur. If there is structural damage, it is called a contusion and is often in the frontal or temporal lobes (shaded areas) of the brain. This bruised nerve tissue may be the site of origin for seizures in post-traumatic epilepsy.

TABLE 20

Characteristics and Treatment of Febrile Seizures in Infants

Simple	Complex
Onset between 1 and 5 years of age	Onset before 1 year of age
Generalized	Focal
Less than 15 minutes long	More than 15 minutes long
Obvious metabolic or infectious disease outside the central nervous system	A history of nonfebrile seizures in family members
No apparent brain damage	Apparent neurologic deficits
No more than one seizure in 24 hours	More than one seizure in 24 hours
Treat by suppressing fever	Treat with antiepileptics

system infection, it is called a simple febrile seizure. This is distinguished from a complex febrile seizure, which lasts more than 15 minutes, has focal features, occurs before 1 year of age, or is associated with a neurologic abnormality or a family history of nonfebrile seizures. The distinction between febrile and nonfebrile is important in determining treatment (Table 20). The simple febrile seizure does not call for antiepileptic therapy; the complex febrile seizure demands it.

Two out of three children with febrile seizures have simple febrile seizures. The likelihood that a child who has had a simple febrile seizure will ever have another one is about 33 percent. Of children exhibiting complex febrile seizures, 10 percent eventually will develop seizures without any associated fever. Of the children with simple febrile seizures, only 2.2 percent will develop convulsions not associated with fevers.

The reason children with simple febrile seizures are not

treated with antiepileptic drugs when high fevers develop is that levels of antiepileptic medication in the blood are achieved too slowly to make a difference when the child is acutely sick, unless the drugs are given intravenously each time a fever appears. The complication rate of intravenous antiepileptic treatment is too high to justify its use with simple febrile seizures.

Children with evidence of central nervous system damage should be started on antiepileptic therapy after their first seizure, even if it was precipitated by a fever. Of children who have febrile seizures on more than three separate occasions, three out of five have a family history of febrile seizures and two out of three have abnormal brain waves. This simply indicates that the child and other affected family members have seizure thresholds low enough that relatively minor stimuli, such as high fevers, are enough to cause seizures. If one child in the family has febrile seizures, the likelihood that its sibling will also have febrile seizures is 10 to 15 percent. If one identical twin has febrile seizures, the likelihood that the other twin will have them is several times greater than this. The more similar the genetic composition and intrauterine experience of two people, the more similar are their susceptibilities to epilepsy.

Occasionally a febrile seizure evolves into a string of seizures rather than just a single convulsion. This string of seizures may turn into an unrelenting and life-threatening condition called status epilepticus. The risk of this is greatest with a child's first febrile seizure. Therefore, any child experiencing his first febrile seizure should be admitted to a hospital for careful observation and evaluation.

A child with febrile seizures may have meningitis—inflammation of the membranes surrounding the brain and spinal cord. Signs of infection in or near the brain in infants can be extremely subtle. A lumbar puncture to check the cerebrospinal fluid may be the only way to determine whether a central nervous system infection is responsible for an infant's seizure disorder. In children under 6 months of age, a life-threatening case of meningitis may show little more than fever and a seizure. In such cases the risks of lumbar puncture are far outweighed by the dangers of not detecting meningitis early in its course.

If treatment of a febrile seizure is warranted, phenobarbital is the drug of choice, at least for the short term. Adverse reactions with this drug, which include irritability, hyperactivity, negativistic behavior, and rashes, occur in about half of all children treated. Despite these disadvantages, phenobarbital is preferred because of its relative safety. Alternative drugs such as sodium valproate can cause liver or pancreatic disease in rare cases. Experience with new drugs is still limited because clinical trials in antiepileptic drug development almost always test drugs in adults long before infants or children are exposed.

Pediatricians and pediatric neurologists do not use phenytoin for febrile seizures because of worries that this drug might slow growth and development in the very young child. Phenytoin does affect calcium metabolism and the availability of folic acid (a vitamin), but it is not obvious that it causes any more problems than phenobarbital. The long experience with and established safety of phenobarbital in the treatment of febrile seizures have made it the drug of choice for most physicians, but this may change as other drugs with fewer side effects are developed. Problems with side effects necessitate stopping the drug in many cases, and as many as one parent in five stops giving the medication without consulting a physician.

Febrile seizures rarely occur in children after age 7. Children 7 or older who develop seizures with high fevers should be investigated even more thoroughly than younger children for tumors and central nervous system infections, both of which require early detection and treatment.

Poisoning

Poisoning is a common cause of seizures in children because they so often swallow items they find lying around, particularly drugs intended for adults, such as aspirin and sleep medications. The poisons likely to cause seizures in children are the same ones that cause seizures in adults. The one exception that particularly affects children is lead. Children ingest lead from soil, paint, plaster, and other materials that adults are not likely to swallow. Toxic levels of lead in the brain usually cause generalized tonic-clonic convulsions. Permanent brain damage from this poison may require long-term antiepileptic treatment.

In most cases of seizure from poisoning, antiepileptic medications are not needed, but if recurrent seizures develop while the poison is being eliminated from the child's body, medication may be required for days or weeks. With every poison, the most important goal is to minimize the damage. Rapid clearance of the poison and close observation of the child during the time it takes to eliminate the poison are essential. In the case of an overdose of a barbiturate, for example, seizures may not occur until the level of barbiturate in the blood begins to drop rapidly.

When children poison themselves with materials or medications they find around the house, their parents often feel terribly guilty and may react by becoming overprotective. It is important for parents to avoid stifling the child with too many limitations and to take a rational approach to protecting the child from potential poisons. Repeated poisonings are common, but the child's extraordinary curiosity is generally more at fault than the parents' carelessness.

Tumors

Brain tumors are a relatively rare cause of seizures in children. Some hereditary disorders, such as tuberous sclerosis (see Chapter 5), produce tumors in the brain during the first months of life; but even with these congenital problems, brain malformations rather than tumors are the usual explanation for seizures. Most childhood tumors occur at the base of the brain in the brainstem or the cerebellum—areas that do not cause seizures when damaged. These tumors may spread to the space overlying the brain and cause irritation that leads to seizures, but this is a later effect. What appears to be a tumor in a very young child should be investigated with a brain biopsy whenever that is feasible. Occasionally a local infection from tuberculosis, parasites, or other agents will masquerade as a mass in the brain. With a biopsy, the appropriate diagnosis and treatment can be determined.

Seizurelike Phenomena

Several behaviors that are easily confused with epilepsy occur in infants and children (Table 21). These abnormalities often involve choking or troubled breathing and may occur only during sleep. The best way to distinguish between seizurelike phenomena and true seizures is to make electroencephalographic (EEG) recordings during the abnormal behavior. Brain waves may change during the episode, but the patterns typical of true seizures, such as rhythmic spikes, sharp waves, or bursts of slow waves (see Chapter 10), do not occur. When the electroencephalographic recording is ambiguous, the setting in which the behavior occurs may be informative. If episodes happen only after an infant resists being fed, for example, the problem is more likely to be gastrointestinal or psychological than neurological.

Breathing Problems

At 6 to 8 weeks of age, some infants develop episodes of choking, during which they seem to have difficulty breathing. This develops without vomiting or any apparent regurgitation of

TABLE 21
Seizurelike Phenomena

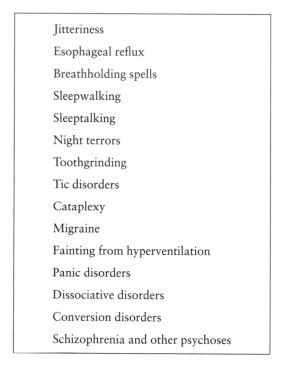

Jitteriness

Esophageal reflux

Breathholding spells

Sleepwalking

Sleeptalking

Night terrors

Toothgrinding

Tic disorders

Cataplexy

Migraine

Fainting from hyperventilation

Panic disorders

Dissociative disorders

Conversion disorders

Schizophrenia and other psychoses

milk or formula, and it is frequently associated with rigid extension or contortions of the arms and legs. The infant may arch its entire body and turn blue. This behavior usually occurs in infants who have poor feeding patterns and whose parents leave them to cry for long periods to get attention. Although no seizure is occurring, the child eventually regurgitates milk or formula into its esophagus and then chokes. Holding the infant while it is fed and for some time afterward is often all that is required to eliminate this disturbing behavior. Without this change in feeding strategy, the regurgitation may persist for months.

Older infants and children may have spells of holding their breath. These spells occur in as much as 5 percent of the general population, and one out of four children with this behavior has another family member with a history of similar spells. These spells generally appear between 6 months and 4 years of age. The child stops breathing for several seconds or minutes and may turn pale or blue. In some infants the problem is an overactive vascular (vasovagal) reflex that causes a marked slowing of the heart rate. In most, it is a behavioral abnormality associated with protracted anger and frustration.

If an overactive vasovagal reflex is responsible, the behavior will abate as the child matures. If the child is holding his breath in reaction to frustration, other behavioral abnormalities are likely to appear as he gets older. Parents can minimize breathholding spells and avoid future behavioral problems by spending more time interacting with the child. They should make sure that their behavior during the spell does not reward breathholding, and they should give consistent incentives for more positive behavior.

Sleep-Related Disorders

Sleepwalking, sleeptalking, and night terrors are not caused by seizures, but some features of each behavior resemble seizures enough to confuse physicians as well as parents. The parents are especially likely to suspect epilepsy if another family member has seizures. Seizures do sometimes occur during sleep and can induce the child to walk, talk, or appear acutely frightened; but seizures usually also appear when a child is awake and produce other signs of abnormal brain activity, such as generalized convulsions, postictal confusion, and premonitory auras.

With both seizures and abnormal sleep behavior, the child does not recall the episode when fully awake. The confusion, irritability, and combativeness exhibited by children during these events support the notion that abnormal brain activity akin to seizures is responsible, but an electroencephalogram will establish that epilepsy is not involved.

Teeth-grinding (bruxism) sometimes arouses concern, but it is so common in the general population that it rarely warrants any investigation. Bedwetting (enuresis), which is usually benign in very young children, may also be a sign of seizures in sleep. Unlike sleepwalking, sleeptalking, and night terrors, bedwetting is usually dismissed by parents as an embarrassing incident rather than a worrisome sign. If the child is entering puberty or late adolescence at the time of the bedwetting, an investigation of the problem is warranted.

Migraine

Migraine headaches in children can cause confused states, memory disturbances, and disorientation, but the pattern of pain and a family history of migraine usually simplify the identification of this problem. Migraine pain is usually on one side of the head and may be centered about or over one eye or temple. The pain lasts minutes to hours and is sometimes associated with nausea and vomiting. Visual changes often warn of an impending migraine.

Some people have migraine fragments—components of the migraine syndrome that appear independently of the headache. Disturbed vision with flickering (scintillation) in the line of sight and blind spots, both of which last minutes to hours, are common migraine fragments. In the classic migraine headaches these phenomena precede the headache and clear completely before the headache starts. As migraine fragments, they come and go without producing headache and raise concerns that the child has sensory seizures.

Migraine appears to involve a disturbance of the vascular supply to the brain. Signs and symptoms vary, depending on which brain arteries are involved. Basilar artery migraine can be especially difficult to diagnose because it involves blood vessels supplying the base of the brain. Symptoms that develop with basilar artery migraine include vertigo, gait disorders, double vision, and vomiting. This type of migraine is uncommon and is more often seen in adolescents and young adults.

Electroencephalographic studies do not help settle the question of whether the problem is migraine or seizures because brain waves are often abnormal with migraine headache. Further confusing the picture is the common report by children and adults that they have headache after their seizures, especially if the seizures are nocturnal. Even a therapeutic trial with an antiepileptic medication will not necessarily distinguish between atypical migraine and focal seizures. Valproate (Depakote) is often effective against both seizure and migraine activity. Other antiepileptic medications are less consistently effective against migraines. A careful assessment of risk factors, clinical course, and family history helps to identify the underlying problem.

Tourette Syndrome and Other Tic Disorders

Involuntary movement disorders, such as facial tics, and peculiar tendencies to vocalize inappropriate sounds or words are occasionally mistaken for seizure activity. These movements or vocalizations may be evidence of Tourette syndrome, a nonepileptic cause of paroxysmal movements and utterances. Making the distinction between Tourette syndrome or a more limited tic disorder and focal seizures is important because the treatments are very different.

Learning and Behavior Problems

Most children who have epilepsy without any other nervous system disease do as well in school as their peers and have no obvious personality disorders. But there are exceptions. Learning disability and behavior problems most commonly appear when there are other neurologic signs in addition to seizures, such as limb weakness or impaired coordination. Overall, children with epilepsy have more behavioral and learning disorders than either healthy children or children with other chronic nonneurologic disorders, such as lung or heart disease. Intermittent disturbance of brain activity certainly plays a role, but parental attitudes and expectations can profoundly influence the child's social and academic performance. Expecting the child to be unable to perform at a level appropriate for his age and intelligence seems to ensure that he will not.

Behavioral problems occur in many different kinds of epilepsy. One of the more obvious is violent or destructive behavior. The type of epilepsy the child has appears to influence whether or not this destructiveness will develop. Children with complex partial and grand mal seizures exhibit slightly more violent behavior than children with more focal seizure disorders. Both boys and girls are more likely to be violent if they have generalized seizures that first develop during late adolescence.

Several types of behavior disorders, not necessarily including violence, are especially prevalent in boys with complex partial seizures. These may involve difficulty in socializing with other children, dealing with failure, participating in family activities, and meeting other common demands of childhood. Destructive behavior is also common in children with the rare generalized nonconvulsive seizures called akinetic seizures. Violent behavior is not common in children with myoclonic seizures. With all types of epilepsy and all types of abnormal behavior considered together, 25 percent of the children with seizure disorders develop psychosocial problems severe enough to justify or require professional attention.

Problems in School

Learning is sometimes a problem for children with epilepsy, but learning disorders can also be exaggerated because of the common misconception that epilepsy and mental retardation are related. For children without mental retardation, whether a learning disability occurs is influenced by the age at which the epilepsy first appears: the later epilepsy develops, the lower the child's risk of learning problems. This is probably because disorders that cause both diffuse brain damage and epilepsy are more likely before 1 year of age than at other ages.

Whatever the reason, children at 9 to 15 years of age with generalized convulsive seizure disorders are significantly less impaired on tests of neuropsychologic performance if their seizures began when they were between 8 and 14 than if they began before age 5. Tasks that require coordination, protracted attention and concentration, complex problem solving, or good memory function are especially difficult for children whose seizures began very early (0–5) or relatively late (14–18).

Children with idiopathic epilepsy, as a group, are much less likely to show impaired cognitive function than are children with symptomatic epilepsy. This is part of the reason for the poorer performance of children who develop epilepsy late in adolescence. These children are less likely to have idiopathic seizures than children whose epilepsy develops at about the time of puberty, and they often have seizures caused by infections and trauma.

Children whose epilepsy develops before age 5 also do more poorly as a group because many of them are impaired by birth asphyxia, intrauterine infections, brain malformations, and other causes of congenital brain damage. Children who are brain-damaged at birth usually develop seizures before their first birthday. The poorer cognitive performance of children whose seizures begin before age 5 is typically not caused by an adverse effect on the brain of the seizures themselves or the antiepileptics used to suppress the seizures but by the underlying condition.

Regardless of their intellectual abilities, children with epilepsy are treated differently in school from other children. Even the most understanding teachers carry their own fears and misconceptions of this disorder. The teacher is often worried about inadvertently causing a seizure, and many parents pass on to the teacher their own inaccurate beliefs. A mother who has seen her child turn blue during a generalized convulsion may tell the teacher that the last seizure nearly killed the child. The epilepsy takes on life-threatening dimensions, and all but the most enlightened teachers will be terrified by the prospect of a seizure occurring in the classroom. The parents' excessive protectiveness is transferred to the classroom, and special treatment may isolate the child from classmates.

If the teacher does not know the child has a seizure disorder, the impact of a seizure at school will be even greater. Children with generalized absence (petit mal) seizures are often accused of daydreaming, since absence attacks are difficult to differentiate from inattentiveness. The child may be disciplined for laziness or disobedience. Teachers unfamiliar with seizure disorders may mistake a generalized convulsion for a fainting spell or a complex partial attack for mental illness or drug use. Even if the teacher can be convinced that the harrowing experience was caused by a relatively benign neurological disorder, the teacher's understandable reluctance to be burdened by the problem will interfere with the child's experience at school.

Teachers frequently describe children with epilepsy as solitary, irritable, uninterested, and unpopular. Much of this behavior may result from the child's recognition that she is different from other children, and from the fact that in school she does not hold the pivotal role she holds at home, even if the teachers are protective. When children with epilepsy lag months or years behind their age group in school, their teachers ascribe this slow advancement to the effects of medication or to parental attitudes. In fact, the problems are often exacerbated by the attitudes of the teachers themselves, who may share the misconception that epilepsy equals mental retardation and so may reduce their expectations of the child.

The relatively poor school adjustment and achievement of children with epilepsy are usually unrelated to any nervous system problem; intelligence tests indicate that they should perform much better than they do. At least part of this underachievement grows out of parents' expectations that the child with epilepsy will do less well in social activities, sports, and scholastic achievement than the child without epilepsy. These expectations are imposed upon the child in a fairly obvious way. Parents seek to excuse the child from sports and other strenuous activities, for example, a maneuver that not only announces the child's problem to classmates and reinforces his sense of being different but also encourages his withdrawal and isolation.

The child's teachers would be helped greatly by an unambiguous statement from the physician of what the child can and cannot do. With the parents' consent, the physician should convey this information directly to the teachers rather than sending it through the parents. If the child is at risk of having seizures, the teacher must be told what to expect and what to do. Despite oppressive parental fears, the real dangers faced by the child who has a seizure in school are minimal. The child should not be kept out of sports and other activities, unless the particular type of epilepsy poses special risks.

Parents' Limited Expectations

Ideally, every parent with a child who has seizures should have an accurate view of what the child's potential is and should help the child to achieve that potential, both at school and at home. Unfortunately, many parents fall short of this ideal. Parents often impose excessive limits on the child with epilepsy, perhaps as an overreaction to their inability to control the seizures. Alternatively, the overprotectiveness may be an attempt to compensate for injuries they imagine they have inflicted on the child. Many parents have a nagging conviction that the child would be fine if they had acted differently. The guilt may take on a religious quality: the parents may see themselves as being punished for a sin or transgression, and so they may feel especially responsible for the affliction visited upon their innocent child.

Of course, some families who limit the goals they set for their children do so out of neglect rather than over-responsibility. The family may have assigned the child the role of cripple and may be reluctant to release the child from that role. Many parents admit that they see their child with epilepsy as a pitiful, unfortunate person who should not be expected to achieve anything. Unfortunately, the child with epilepsy, like any child, incorporates his parents' opinions about himself. If the parents believe that the child cannot achieve anything substantial, the child soon believes it too. Many children with epilepsy have inappropriately low aspirations and become very dependent in interpersonal relationships.

Children with epilepsy often have trouble developing relationships with other children. They tend to be isolated from their peers but inordinately dependent upon their mothers. This failure to socialize develops partly because of parental restrictions. The parents lack confidence that the child can manage outside the family if a seizure occurs, and a seizure can occur at any time. The child adopts this parental attitude and clings to the family.

To allow the child to grow into a normal, capable adult, parents must be willing to involve the child with the world outside the home. Recreational camps, extramural school activities, and other well-structured settings in which the child can mix with other children and adults will make him or her more flexible and resourceful even if the parents have trouble shedding their own limited expectations. Parents should encourage their child to participate in such activities.

Behavioral Effects of Antiepileptic Drugs

Treatment of epilepsy is no more complicated and no less successful in children than in adults, but some adverse reactions that develop in children on antiepileptic drugs rarely appear in adults. Some of the difficulty with learning and behavior observed in children with epilepsy may be an effect of their antiepileptic medication.

Phenobarbital is being used less each year as alternative antiepileptics are introduced, but many physicians still use it to treat generalized seizures in childhood. One of its side effects is hyperactivity. Although phenobarbital is a sedative in adults, it may arouse children to excessive and sometimes destructive behavior. Children taking phenobarbital are often inattentive, irritable, aggressive, and tearful. Primidone (Mysoline), a drug partly metabolized to phenobarbital and sometimes used to treat complex partial seizures, can have many of the same side effects as phenobarbital. Hyperactivity may be so disruptive to the child and his family that other antiepileptic drugs must be tried until a more suitable drug is found.

Generalized absence (petit mal) seizures are usually treated with ethosuximide (Zarontin), which occasionally causes irritability directly or by interfering with sleep. Children on ethosuximide have a special susceptibility to night terrors, frightening images that occur during sleep and awaken the child. Myoclonic and other types of epilepsy that do not respond to conventional antiepileptics are often treated with clonazepam (Klonopin), which can cause withdrawn behavior, mood swings, and auditory hallucinations.

Sometimes behavioral problems appear in children with epilepsy that are unrelated to either the medication or the seizures themselves. For many of these children, temper tantrums, poor tolerance of frustration, and hyperactivity improve with age rather than with any specific treatment. Children with behavioral problems that do not respond to changes in medication and do not improve with age often have obvious structural damage to the brain. In fact, structural brain damage and intellectual impairment resulting from undiscovered brain damage are more frequently responsible for hyperactivity and destructiveness in children than is any social factor.

Conflicts within the Family

Epilepsy in a child unavoidably disturbs relationships in the family. This disturbance grows out of the child's self-image as well as the way the rest of the family sees the child. From an early age the child with epilepsy, rather than developing a sense of competence, experiences an inability to control his own body. In many families, this fear and insecurity are magnified in the exchange between child and parents. Both the child and the parents are uncomfortably aware of their inability to control the epilepsy. Parents may have excessive concern for the child's well-being, may strenuously deny the problem, or may simply reject him because of his chronic disorder. Often the parents' feelings toward the child involve an element of shame. This embarrassment over having a chronically ill child is rarely overt, but it is apparent to the child.

Many parents fail to seek authoritative information on their child's seizure disorder or to discuss it with their child in a frank way. The parents are frightened by the seizures and often have no idea of what to do when one occurs even if they have discussed them with a physician. More than half never read anything about epilepsy, but they do gather considerable hearsay from friends and relatives. This fosters misconceptions that may be damaging to the child.

Because many parents do not understand the causes and consequences of their child's epilepsy, they are most comfortable raising the child according to arbitrary and highly restrictive guidelines. The more inflexible the parents are, the more of a problem the epilepsy is likely to be. Even seizure control is related to parental attitudes. Children with autocratic parents have poorer seizure control on antiepileptic drugs than do children with less restrictive parents. Children do best, at least in terms of seizure control, in families that allow them a normal level of independence and discipline.

Manipulation of Parents by Children

Parents usually treat children with epilepsy the way they would treat any sick child. The problem with this approach is that most illnesses are transient, whereas epilepsy continues for years or a lifetime. Unless the parents are unusually well-informed, they are likely to worry that they will inadvertently make the epilepsy worse. Even if they know that their every action and remark will not significantly affect the disorder, each severe attack will stir up the notion that the child might have fared better if they had behaved differently.

Children quickly realize that parental fears and guilt are easily played upon. Any attempts to discipline the child can be subverted by the threat that such treatment will cause a seizure. This manipulation of the parents aggravates an already difficult family situation and evokes much resentment among parents and siblings, a resentment that is often not recognized by the people experiencing it.

A child with severely disabling seizures imposes restrictions on the family that may make the child a virtual tyrant over the family. All family activities may be fashioned around the child's limitations. Parents who are angry at these limitations may feel guilty because of this anger. In their guilt, the parents may give in to the epileptic child's every whim, always believing they want to do only what is best for the child.

The child who is frightened of traveling may become ill whenever a trip is planned. The parents may worry about what effect travel actually has on the child, but they cannot help resenting the limitations placed on them by the neurologic condition. To avoid conflict, the parents may check with the child before making plans. The child, frustrated by being unable to control the epilepsy, finds that he has considerable control over family activities. He may even pretend to have seizures at various times as a way of gaining control over circumstances in his own life (see Chapter 10).

A balance must be struck between the needs of the person with epilepsy and the needs of the entire family. To minimize the likelihood of a power struggle, the parents must be consistent and fair. The child must be shown that intimidation will not work and that illness is not beneficial. When a trip is planned, it should be carried out. If the child seems to be unable to participate in a family activity, then alternative arrangements should be made for her care; the family should not give up the activity. The entire family should not be governed by the whim or illness of the child with epilepsy, and the child should be able to rely upon the parents' judgment when an activity is planned.

Many children discover that they can trigger seizures with certain stimuli, and usually they discover it at about the same time they discover the power they can exert in the family by having seizures. One young woman whose complex partial seizures were not diagnosed until she was well over 20 years old recalled amusing herself as a child by rotating a mayonnaise jar in the refrigerator as fast as she could. The rotating pattern would bring on visual hallucinations, including a hula dancer, that she found fascinating. These were sensory seizures that she induced in herself by moving the jar, and she later developed complex partial seizures with visual hallucinations as part of the aura.

This particular young woman did not tell her parents about these hallucinations and never considered them at all peculiar until questioned about the different types of hallucinations she developed as an adult. But sometimes children who can bring on their own seizures find themselves in a powerful bargaining position in the family. They have the option of simply becoming sick if the adults do not do what they want. They can make seizures occur at very inopportune times if they choose. This behavior will bring the most unbending parent to compromise. The main disadvantage of this maneuver is that the child in the sick role is excluded from many activities that he might enjoy.

To minimize this type of activity, it is important that the child is not rewarded for it. A seizure, real or otherwise, should not consume all of a parent's energies. The spouse and the other children have equally legitimate claims on the parent's attention and affection, and they should not be neglected. Ascribing too much importance to seizures and giving them too much attention encourage the child to exploit them.

Parental Control of the Child's Life

Parents are often frightened by their lack of control over seizures, and some are constantly terrified that the child will die during a seizure while they stand by helplessly. How they react to this impotence varies. A few parents simply deny that their child has any problem at all and insist that the child could be like any other children if he wanted to be. When parents ignore all the precautions that are appropriate for a child with seizures, they may claim they are following the physician's instructions. If the physician uses euphemisms to refer to the epilepsy, the parents may take this lack of frankness as evidence that the problem is not epilepsy or, alternatively, that epilepsy is too terrible to discuss forthrightly. Some parents avoid telling the child what his problem is and pretend that the medication is a vitamin or a pill for a less serious disorder. Whatever attitude the family members take early on is likely to harden as the condition continues.

Denial of the problem is less common than overattention to it. Parents often react to their inability to control seizures by extending their influence and protection over inappropriate areas of the child's life. One-third of parents of children with epilepsy believe that the children require constant supervision, even after the seizures have been completely controlled for months or years. Parents encourage passivity in these children and discourage self-reliance and initiative. Eating habits, friendships, travel patterns, and play may all be regulated with an inappropriate and unproductive strictness.

The struggle to control the child is disguised as a wish to protect him. All excitement is banned because of the risk of seizures. No opportunities to fail are allowed, even if that failure will be instructive. Any activity that makes the parent nervous is forbidden because it may cause seizures. Exaggerating their legitimate concern that a seizure may occur in a dangerous situation, the parents may constantly monitor and restrict the child's activities.

Even when parents' efforts to limit the child's activities are successful, they are usually only temporarily so. Restricting the child's autonomy backfires in most cases because the child eventually either rebels against all rules or becomes passive and dependent upon the restrictive parents. In early childhood the most common reaction is passivity and withdrawal. The child interacts with parents and siblings as little as possible and accepts parental decisions without resistance. This response to excessive restriction is often misconstrued by the parents as an effect of the epilepsy itself or of the medication. It is important to recognize the behavior for what it is, if only to minimize problems when the child becomes more independent. Unfortunately, a well-established pattern of dependence upon their parents leaves many children ill-prepared to manage the epilepsy and to take responsibility for other aspects of their lives when they become adults.

In some families the child with epilepsy becomes an excuse to keep the parents' marriage together. The parents may have little bond besides the child's dependence upon them; and if one of them wants the marriage to continue, the child's dependence may become an indispensable element in that parent's strategy. Any attempts by the child to be independent will undermine it. Thus the parent treats the child as helpless regardless of his of her real abilities and needs. The couple avoid dealing with their own conflicts by focusing their resentment and frustration on the child's chronic problem. The family becomes centered upon the child simply to survive.

Even when the person with seizures is not exploited to stabilize the family, the epilepsy itself lends a distinctive character to the way the family functions. Families with an epileptic child are more disciplined than other families. This is true even when the child has been seizure-free for more than six months. Problems are solved in an efficient, albeit tyrannical, manner. The hierarchy is much more evident and rigid in these families than in families without epileptic children, and this hierarchy is not quickly disassembled after its organizing influence is no longer needed. The mother assumes an inordinately dominant position if she is primarily responsible for the child. Apparently this rigid family structure not only serves the child's need to be protected and supervised but also protects the family from the disruptive effects of the disorder.

This rigid pattern of family interactions can limit the child's ability to cope outside the family. By sheltering the child from failure, the parents keep him from becoming independent. The most routine tasks, such as preparing food, shopping, and choosing clothing, may be taken over by the parents in the unspoken belief that the child could not do them without failing. The suspicion that the child is not competent to take on routine tasks may be accurate in some cases, but parents who do not give the child a chance to be responsible for such activities ensure that he will never become competent.

The Adolescent with Epilepsy

Epilepsy presents several new problems in adolescence. The crucial issues at this time of life are independence, identity, and conformity, all of which are complicated by epilepsy and its treatment. In the United States, part of the independence that comes with adolescence is getting a driver's license. Many adolescents deny that they have epilepsy if admitting it is likely to prevent them from driving.

Part of denying the epilepsy is not taking medication, a practice the adolescent usually identifies with overbearing parents anyway. Peers tend to question any drug-taking and treat someone they know to have epilepsy as different. Medication and visits to the physician become a focus for issues of control between adolescents and their parents. Adolescents often refuse to take medication when control is incomplete but seizures are not totally disabling. The apparent ineffectiveness of the medication makes the adolescent more inclined to resent attempts to regulate his life, a life that is disrupted by the threat of seizures.

Adolescents with relatively minor seizure disorders may have worse social adjustment than those with severe epilepsy because they feel more annoyed than burdened by the seizures and more burdened than helped by the antiepileptic medications. They see themselves repeatedly frustrated in trying to have the lifestyle of their peers, a lifestyle independent of medication and of many restrictions on their activities. Adolescents who have more frequent or more severe seizures usually are more cooperative in following medication recommendations and activity restrictions.

Karen, a high school student who had concealed her seizures from her friends for years, was determined to try out for the swimming team even though she had never been an avid swimmer, because all her friends were on the team. Her mother forbade her from swimming, but Karen ignored this restriction even though she knew she faced a real danger. She told her mother that she knew what she was doing, and that if she was going to die, she was at least going to die happy. She did not drown, and her seizure disorder certainly did not make swimming impossible. But her main reason for joining the team was to demonstrate to her friends that she needed to observe no precautions. This recklessness had developed in opposition to her family's excessive cautiousness.

Finding a way to cope with the seizure disorder is so

difficult for most parents that they seem unable to adjust their strategies as the child gets older. Emily's mother insisted that if Emily would only do what she was told repeatedly to do, she would not have recurrent seizures. The mother blamed recent seizures on Emily's erratic sleeping schedule, poor diet, excessive socializing, and rowdy friends. With obvious sincerity, the concerned mother told Emily's physician, "I've told her many times that I disapprove of her behavior." The daughter was 34 years old, married, with children of her own, but her mother still treated her the same way she had when Emily developed seizures at 5 years of age. Emily resented her mother's prying and described her mother as an ever-critical, disruptive force that she could not escape. The mother blamed the seizures on whatever behavior she disapproved of and took her complaints to her son-in-law when her daughter refused to listen.

This is an example of a common problem: many parents treat their child with epilepsy in the same way for decades. Such inflexibility leads to a progressive alienation of the person with epilepsy from the family. This pattern also contributes to the isolation felt by many adults with epilepsy.

Drug and Alcohol Abuse

In a culture prone to drug abuse, the epileptic adolescent's unlimited access to controlled substances can provide an easy route to popularity. The sale or free distribution of barbiturates by adolescents with epilepsy is enough of a problem in some cities to require highly regulated access to these medications. Some of these adolescents themselves abuse the drugs; after years of resisting parental pressure to take the medication, they experiment with excessive doses of antiepileptics.

Regular monitoring of blood levels will help detect much of this abuse, but the best approach is simply to switch to antiepileptic drugs without any resale value or well-recognized potential for abuse, such as phenytoin (Dilantin), carbamazepine (Tegretol), lamotrigine (Lamictal), gabapentin (Neurontin), or valproate (Depakote).

Alcohol and other drugs used for recreation alter the metabolism of antiepileptic drugs. Adolescents exhibit as little judgment in using alcohol, barbiturates, and other intoxicants as adults do. Cocaine and methamphetamine lower the seizure threshold. Excessive alcohol or barbiturate intake makes a person more vulnerable to seizures, which occur when the level of alcohol or barbiturate in the blood falls. If the adolescent has concealed the drug abuse, his parents may take him to the doctor in extrme anxiety over the recurrence of seizures.

Abuse of drugs of any kind is more severe in families where adults have their own addictions. A child who is ordered not to drink alcohol by a parent who drinks every day is likely to ignore the instruction. Parents who are dependent upon sedatives or other types of relaxants are poor models for children who must be careful in their use of drugs.

Prognosis

Even before antiepileptic drugs were discovered, many seizure disorders disappeared within months or years of their appearance. This is still true. Of the people who consult a doctor within a year of the appearance of episodes that are thought to be seizures, as many as 85 percent have spontaneous remission of their disorder. This drops to 50 percent for people who are not seen by a physician until the episodes have persisted for more than a year; but this simply means that if the problem is epilepsy and the epilepsy is going to disappear on its own, it will often do so within a year of its appearance.

Different types of seizures exhibit different tendencies to remit. Generalized absence (petit mal) seizures often abate late in adolescence and leave the affected person with no signs of brain damage. Infantile spasms, in contrast, usually are associated with devastating neurologic problems in children who have this type of seizure disorder.

Antiepileptics have not substantially affected the remission rates of different types of epilepsy. What they have affected is the harm done by the seizure disorders. Aside from the obvious social toll to the person and the family, an active seizure disorder poses real medical risks. Frequent seizures in children may even contribute to a deterioration in their cognitive abilities, not necessarily because of brain damage but simply because of the restraints on cognitive development imposed by frequent seizures. The risk of premature death is also increased, because children with seizures face a higher risk of accidents than children without them.

Should a First Seizure Be Treated?

Aside from the controversy surrounding the treatment of febrile seizures, real questions exist about whether a single seizure of any type justifies treatment. In children many seizure disorders occur repeatedly before they are even suspected. The initial absence attack or myoclonic seizure usually goes unnoticed or is ascribed to fatigue, inattention, or restlessness. These seizures demand treatment when they are finally recognized. Seizures that occur only when the child is asleep also require investigation and treatment. Nocturnal seizures are just as serious as those that occur when the child is awake and active. More controversial is what to do for a child who has his first grand mal, focal sensory, focal motor, or complex partial seizure.

The risk of subsequent seizures can be estimated according to the cause of the seizure, the incidence of epilepsy in the family, and the electroencephalographic pattern observed after the child has recovered from the seizure, but this estimate is not a guarantee that seizures will or will not recur. The child's age at the initial seizure, the type of seizure observed, and any neurologic abnormalities that might be found on first examining the child do not indicate the risk of recurrence of the seizure. Even if the first seizure episode is status epilepticus, later seizures may not develop once that first episode has passed. Of people who have an idiopathic seizure and epileptic siblings, 35 percent have another seizure within four months.

Abnormal brain wave patterns may persist for years without any further actual seizures, but a generalized spike and slow wave pattern on the electroencephalogram when a person has fully recovered from his first seizure does indicate a high likelihood of recurrent seizures. Half of children with this electroencephalographic abnormality will have another seizure within 18 months. If spikes appear over the central temporal area, the risk of recurrent seizures may be even greater. When the electroencephalogram is normal or has nonspecific abnormalities, the likelihood that an idiopathic seizure will be followed by a second seizure within two years is only 14 percent.

If the initial seizure follows a significant head injury, the risk of a second seizure within 20 months is 46 percent. Seizures that can be related to nervous system problems other than head trauma will recur within 20 months in 28 percent of cases. The risk of recurrence is not substantially affected by the prescription of antiepileptic medication, but this may be because people who have had only one seizure often stop taking the medication after a few weeks.

Long-term Treatment

Both parents and children often ask if the drugs used to control the seizures can be stopped. The side effects of the antiepileptic drug may interfere with the child's social acceptance, and so the affected person hopes to discontinue the drugs as early as possible. Some types of childhood seizure disorders are clearly self-limiting. For example, by the end of adolescence the child with benign Rolandic seizures of child-hood will be seizure-free. With this type of seizure disorder, the family can be told not only that the medication can be stopped but also when. Obviously, if a child has poorly con-trolled seizures while on antiepileptics, it is not appropriate to stop the drugs. The true dilemma arises when a child's sei-zures have been completely controlled for several years. For-tunately there are empirical guidelines for deciding what to do.

If there is no apparent explanation for the seizures, even if the person has focal neurologic abnormalities, the risk of sei-zures recurring is 26 percent once three seizure-free years have passed. If the person had earlier neurologic injury from, say, meningitis or a head injury, the risk of recurrence goes up to 34 percent after three seizure-free years.

After four years without seizures on antiepileptic medica-tion, a child has a 72 percent chance of remaining seizure-free for decades if he stops taking the antiepileptic medications. Of the 28 percent whose seizures recur after going off the drugs, 85 percent will have the relapse within the first five years and 56 percent will have the relapse in the first year. The risk of re-lapse is greatest if the child had several years of poor seizure control before control was finally achieved, if there is un-equivocal central nervous system damage associated with the seizures, if the child had jacksonian or other types of focal motor seizures, or if the child has had more than one type of seizure. Children with a history of a febrile seizure followed by a nonfebrile seizure also run a substantial risk of recurrent seizures when medication is discontinued.

With certain types of seizures, spontaneous remission is very likely. Of children whose electroencephalograms show no abnormality except in the brain waves arising from the oc-cipital lobe, 48 percent will be seizure-free by the time they reach 9 years of age. The actual number of seizures the person had before control was achieved does not affect the likelihood that he will remain seizure-free without medication. The age of the child when medication is stopped is also not important in determining the likelihood of remission, unless the seizures resisted control for several years before the child became seizure-free. The age at onset of the epilepsy, the sex of the child, and a family history of epilepsy also do not affect the likelihood of remaining seizure-free, even though some of these factors do influence the likelihood that a single seizure will develop into epilepsy.

Once a seizure disorder has become established and seizures have been controlled with antiepileptic drugs, relapse is not more frequent in children with persistently abnormal electroencephalograms, so these cannot be used as an indication of the probability of remission. The people with the best chance of remaining seizure-free without medication after four years of complete control are those with generalized, that is, grand mal and petit mal, seizures. Although grand mal seizures have always been viewed with the most horror by the parents of children with epilepsy, they actually have a relatively good prognosis.

Mortality

Premature death in children with epilepsy is a preoccupation of many parents, but the data do not support this worry. When the first seizure occurs, many parents believe that their child is dying. This panic hardly subsides as the seizures become more routine. There are certain progressive diseases of the nervous system that cause seizures and are lethal during childhood, but the seizures associated with these diseases are not the cause of death. Even among people whose epilepsy starts in adolescence, death rates do not rise above those of the general population.

The excess mortality that does occur in young people who have seizures independent of progressive brain disease is caused by status epilepticus, accidents, and suicide (see Chapter 10). Suicide attempts are not particularly common in children or adolescents, although by failing to take medication a person may inadvertently risk death. Accidents are very common in epileptic children and adolescents, but in fatal accidents it is often impossible to determine if the epilepsy or antiepileptic medication played any role.

Strategies for Managing Childhood Seizure Disorders

Most children with epilepsy have normal intelligence, unimpaired growth, and conventional expectations. If a child's epilepsy is caused by a serious nervous system disturbance, this will usually be evident before or shortly after the appearance of the epilepsy. If it is a treatable condition, the seizures may remit when it is corrected. If it is untreatable, the child's prognosis will be determined by the problem causing the seizures, not by the seizures themselves.

Some types of epilepsy are not usually persistent: febrile seizures more often than not are benign and require no treatment other than management of the fever and the infection causing the fever. Some types of nonfebrile childhood seizures, such as Rolandic seizures, are also benign and will disappear as the child matures. Before initiating treatment for any seizure, the physician must establish that the child actually does have epilepsy. Several benign conditions, such as breathholding spells and migraine, may resemble epilepsy, but careful neurologic assessment will determine which children have epilepsy and which do not.

Those children who do have epilepsy face a variety of social problems. They may be singled out at home and at school as distinctly different from their peers, and this assessment often becomes self-fulfilling. This stigmatizing of the child with epilepsy can be minimized if the parents and other family members have a clear idea of what the child can and cannot do.

Abilities, rather than disabilities, should be emphasized. Career goals should be fostered with as little reference to the seizure disorder as possible. An older child hoping to be a jet pilot should obviously be informed of the impossibility of this line of work for a person with epilepsy, but very few fields are so inflexible.

Problems that develop because of the epilepsy should be discussed, but not obsessively; and honesty inside and outside the family should be encouraged. Fantasies about epilepsy, which occur in even the most sophisticated families, are counterproductive and must be explored and discarded. Blaming the epilepsy on some member of the family is especially disruptive. Accusations of blame are a poorly disguised attempt by the family members making the accusations to dissociate themselves from the problem.

Many of the conflicts that easily develop in a family with an epileptic child can be avoided if all family members recognize that the child's epilepsy increases the family's stress load. Power struggles between the affected child and other members of the family should be identified and stopped before manipulation becomes a way of life. The child should be allowed to face the usual challenges of childhood and to fail. She has nothing to be embarrassed about or ashamed of and should be treated accordingly by her parents.

As the child matures, relationships between the epileptic child and other members of his family must be especially flexible. Maturation does not necessarily resolve the problems caused by epilepsy, and in fact it may present new ones. Adolescents with epilepsy are often just as impaired by the seizure disorder as they were in childhood, but they are much less cooperative.

One way to minimize the antagonism that appears between epileptic adolescents and their parents is gradually to give adolescents more responsibility for their own activities and for managing their seizures. The older child or teenager should be encouraged to be responsible for taking medication and ob-serving reasonable precautions. He should be allowed to deal directly with physicians. By gradually giving the child more responsibility for managing his disorder, parents may ensure that when their adolescent is most insistent on being inde-pendent, he is adequately prepared to be independent.

Chapter Seven

Growing Up with an Epileptic Parent

Carlos was born a year after his father developed epilepsy. The father's seizures were totally disabling, so he was usually at home, and Carlos was often present during seizures. When Carlos started crawling, he treated the seizures as a game. He would laugh during the falls and convulsions and even climb onto his father during some of the attacks. This amusement passed within a few months, and by his first birthday the child would cry when a seizure occurred and be agitated for hours afterward. Despite his obvious discomfort with the attacks, the child stayed near his father during most of the day. His father noticed that Carlos was almost always with him when he had a seizure and always there when he awoke from a seizure.

Carlos started talking when he was about a year old, and his most common phrase was "He's okay," which he would say to his mother after his father had recovered from a seizure. During the early postictal period, the father would open his eyes and look around with obvious confusion. Carlos would stare at his father's face until the eyes opened and then announce, "He's okay, he's okay." When Carlos began speaking in fuller sentences, he would run to his mother when his father showed any signs of developing a seizure and tell her, "Daddy is sick again."

By 18 months Carlos could imitate the seizures with extraordinary accuracy. He would reenact the facial expressions and limb postures that preceded a convulsion. He would fall to the ground, roll his eyes, and exhibit both the tonic (spastic) and clonic (rhythmically contracting) phases of his father's seizures. This became a way to amuse friends; Carlos would imitate seizures at parties for his playmates. At one party a child was frightened by the seizure and told his mother, "I think Carlos is dead." Carlos opened his eyes and said, "I'm not dead. I'm just having a seizure."

Carlos also used his ability to imitate seizures to get attention. On a shopping trip with his parents, he saw a mechanical horse he wanted to ride. When his parents refused to let him get on the horse, he had a pseudoseizure. Other shoppers, seeing him thrashing about on the floor, asked his apparently unconcerned parents if they could help. When one passerby demanded that the parents help the child with his seizure, Carlos announced, "I'm not having a real seizure. I just want to play on the horse." At the end of every pseudoseizure, Carlos would open his eyes and say, "I'm okay. I'm okay." His parents bought him a toy telephone, and he often pretended to call his father's doctor. His parents would overhear him saying, "Hello, Doctor Rothman. My daddy is okay today."

Whether parents try to conceal their seizures from their children or explain to the children that the epilepsy is not a sign of serious disease, children are usually aware of their parents' problem and feel anxious about it. The anxiety is apparent whether the child is a toddler or an adolescent. As was obvious in Carlos's case, knowing about the parent's epilepsy from the beginning does not necessarily make it less distressing.

How the young child understands the neurologic disorder is obviously influenced by the parents' attitudes. If the parents offer no explanation for what is happening, the child may develop an explanation that blames himself for causing the seizures. Part of the child's reaction is a fear of being abandoned; this is more of a preoccupation for toddlers and young children than for adolescents and young adults. Older children and adolescents worry about how their peers will view the parent's disorder. The notion that the epilepsy is hereditary or indicates a hereditary mental defect is pervasive enough that many children will conceal their parent's problem. Many children of epileptic parents worry that they will develop epilepsy.

Learning about Epilepsy

Carlos learned about his father's seizures by seeing them occur. The postictal confusion, frequent injuries, and protracted fatigue associated with the seizures became as familiar to him as any element of his father's daily routine. Why he perceived these episodes as dangerous is not clear. His parents had married at about the same time as the first appearance of the seizures. Within a few months of the marriage it was obvious that the husband's episodic confusion was caused by a seizure disorder. The wife's resolve to have a successful marriage was unshaken by the revelation that her husband had epilepsy. Over the years she dealt with seizures calmly and consistently. She was not outwardly anxious during the attacks, and she allowed the child to watch the attacks so that he could see that nothing permanent was happening to his father. Carlos was an only child, so his anxiety was not based upon the reaction of older siblings. Friends and relatives who were present during some attacks did become very agitated, and this may have suggested to the child that something terrible was happening.

Although most people with epilepsy get their information about the disorder from their physicians, and their spouses often ask the physician questions, the children of an epileptic parent usually find out whatever they know about the disorder from one of their parents. The information they get is often distorted. The person with epilepsy usually does not absorb much of what he is told by his physician at the time of diagnosis, and he may be reluctant to ask detailed questions later, after months or years have passed. Basic questions such as "Is this epilepsy?" or "Can this be treated?" will be asked and answered over and over. Obviously, patients who are dazed by the news that they have a chronic illness are poor sources of information for their children. The parent without epilepsy is rarely better prepared to explain the problem to the children. The parents may use ambiguous terms to describe the disorder, such as drop attacks, apoplexy, blackouts, spells, or nervousness.

Many children are unaware that their parent has a seizure disorder until they witness an attack. When the child then is told that the problem has existed for years, he is likely to be skeptical and untrusting. Knowing that he has not been told the truth about his parent's health in the past, he has little reason to believe he is now being given all the facts. Without a reliable source of information in the family, the child will learn about the disorder from peers, television programs, and publications. These sources give the child no opportunity to clarify what his parent's particular problem is. Epilepsy is usually portrayed as a single entity, rather than as a collection of disorders that vary from person to person. The child may get the impression that his parent's condition is much more serious and dangerous than it really is.

The child is at the greatest disadvantage if he is told nothing about the parent's disorder. Not only must he gather information from unreliable sources, but he must also search for explanations for why his parents are not willing to talk about the problem. The 7-year-old neighbor of a middle-aged man who had recently developed seizures asked if the man "would have to be put to sleep." The child had had a dog that had been put to sleep because of epilepsy, and as far as she knew, this was the way to treat the disorder. This type of information is what the child of an epileptic parent must contend with if the parents do not discuss the problem in terms the child can understand. If the parents make it clear that epilepsy is a topic the family can discuss, the misinformation passed along by other children can be brought home and considered there.

Many children who are not fully informed about their parent's disorder will assume that insanity or a lethal illness such as a brain tumor is causing the trouble. Warren, a middle-aged physician with complex partial seizures, never told any of his four children that he had a seizure disorder. He insisted, "This does not affect them in any way. There's no reason to burden them with this." He maintained that, despite disruptive attacks, none of his family other than his wife and no one that he worked with suspected that he had epilepsy. Subsequently he had a seizure while driving with his youngest children in the car. They were unhurt but terrified.

Still insisting that knowing about the epilepsy would only frighten them, Warren avoided any discussion about the accident and continued to drive as if this posed no danger for him or his children. Later he had another seizure while driving, and this one caused an accident. His youngest daughter, who was with him at the time of the accident, refused to ride with him after that, although he assured her that nothing was wrong. His children, forced to guess what the problem was, found their assumptions frightening enough to insist that their father not be responsible for their safety.

Fear of Abandonment

Seizures in a parent are frightening to children of any age, but young children have some very special fears. The most obvious concern of the young child is that the parent may abandon him. Whether the child actually witnesses the parent's attacks or only witnesses the responses of other family members, he invariably worries about losing a parent.

The child may react to this fear in several ways. Carlos became obsessed with his father's well-being and constantly monitored it. Another child, Robert, reacted with more alarm to his father's seizures, but also took on the role of monitor for the family. Robert was 3 when his father's seizures, a result of surgery the father had undergone before Robert was born, became poorly controlled. Over the course of a year Robert witnessed several seizures. Each time he cried uncontrollably and could not be comforted. After a seizure episode, he would stay awake most of the night. Several times he asked his mother, "Is Daddy going to die?" Despite reassurances from both of his parents, he insisted, "I'm sleeping with my daddy." Both parents described Robert as the "closest of all the children to his father." After his parents were in bed, Robert routinely knocked on the bedroom door and asked, "Daddy, are you okay?"

Loss of a Dependable Parent

Children may assume considerable responsibility for the epileptic parent, but they too need someone to rely on. They sometimes shift their dependence from the adult with seizures to other family members. Karina, the teenage daughter of a woman who developed epilepsy late in life, showed considerable concern about her mother's health, but she relied on other members of her family for advice and assistance. Her mother developed seizures just as Karina was about to take a trip abroad, and Karina was confused about whether to go. Her maternal aunt and grandfather insisted that she go. Over the next few years Karina continued to turn to her mother's sister for the kind of guidance that would ordinarily be provided by a parent. She remained quite attached to her mother, but she described her mother's illness as if she, rather than her mother, had suffered an injury. She said, "It was the worst thing that ever happened to me."

The shift away from dependence on the epileptic parent is

probably reinforced by this feeling of injury. Karina's belief that the epilepsy was an injury to her is not at all unusual. David, an 11-year-old boy who did not know about his mother's lifelong generalized seizures until he witnessed one, became hysterical during the seizure. He hid and cried, and when his mother recovered he complained to her that it was not fair to him for her to be sick. He spoke of her illness as if it were terminal, insisting, "You can't be that sick. I didn't know you were so sick." His mother's epilepsy was actually easily controlled, and her seizure occurred only because of a lapse in medication combined with alcohol abuse. David felt that he had been tricked by not being told about her disease, and he refused to believe it was not lethal.

David's 14-year-old sister took the episode more stoically, but later in the day surprised her mother with the announcement, "You can't have this. You can't do this to me." In keeping with the family tradition of not discussing the epilepsy, both children refused to discuss the episode further and rejected the proposal that they visit the neurologist's office to have their questions answered.

The parent's seizures are a divisive element in some families. If the child is asked to watch the parent with epilepsy and report his or her behavior to the other parent, the family may split into two camps. The daughter of a middle-aged man with seizures was in the car when her father had an episode of altered consciousness and drove off the road. Because he did not want to give up driving, the girl lied to her mother about the accident. She insisted that her father had not had a seizure, even though she knew that a seizure had endangered both her and her father. By covering up for her father, she established herself as an adversary to her mother, who sought to protect her husband and children by denying him activities he enjoyed.

Whether the child takes on responsibility for the epileptic parent or relies on another adult, the child does not consider the parent a dependable source of guidance and comfort. If the child learns about the seizures after the parents have concealed them for years, the parents lose credibility. The notion that a parent's seizure disorder is of no concern to the children is apparently not shared by the children once they discover the disorder.

Fears of Developing Epilepsy

Children of epileptic parents often fear that they will develop the disorder when they get older. This concern is evident whether the affected parent has idiopathic epilepsy or seizures secondary to a structural brain injury. When the fear is appropriate, the child may exhibit an extraordinary level of denial. When Myra first developed seizures in her teens, she refused to believe she had a permanent disorder, even though her father, brother, and grandfather had epilepsy. Despite having generalized convulsions with loss of consciousness at dangerous times, she refused to take antiepileptic medications, insisting that she would grow out of the problem. She continued to have brief episodes of confusion for several years, but consistently denied that they were related to epilepsy. She frequently lost personal items, including her wallet, and often could not remember how she had arrived home. When her problem was revealed to her father's neurologist, she stopped accompanying her parents to the doctor's office.

Recommendations

The children of people with epilepsy show a remarkably limited range of reactions to the disorder. Regardless of the age of the child, the least disruptive approach for the parents to take seems to be full disclosure. Unless the child is exceedingly unperceptive, he will notice the parent's altered consciousness, abnormal movements, or other seizure phenomena. If the seizures are fully controlled, the parent's chronic dependence on medication will arouse suspicion that a medical problem is involved. It is unrealistic to expect children to ask questions about a problem their parents refuse to discuss. Even when the problem is finally out in the open, children will still tend to stick to the pattern the family developed over the years. That is, they will avoid the topic with the same fervor exhibited by their parents.

Parents who are "found out" because they have a seizure are compromised in two respects in the eyes of their children. They are no longer physically reliable, and they lose their credibility. The child assumes that an illness justifying such secrecy must be grave. And the parent's reassurances that it is not serious are not believed, because the parent has been found untrustworthy.

Frank discussion of the neurologic problem and its treatment can avoid the distrust and resentment that usually develop when the parents try to conceal epilepsy. Because parents may be burdened by their own misconceptions about the disorder, they would be wise to involve a medical or mental health professional in at least some of the family discussions.

Chapter Eight

Siblings and the Extended Family

Witnessing a seizure can be a frightening experience for the brother, sister, grandparent, or other relative of a person with epilepsy. The distress of relatives who see someone in the family have a seizure or who simply learn of the epilepsy often contributes to the isolation of the person with the disorder. Relatives are subject to the same prejudices and misconceptions as anyone else. Finding out that a family member has epilepsy does not correct these misconceptions and may even solidify what had been vague concerns and fears.

When epilepsy occurs in a child, it may interfere with the development of constructive relationships between the child and her brothers and sisters, who often resent the special treatment and considerable attention directed toward the epileptic child. The adult who develops epilepsy also inevitably faces some deterioration in family ties. Why this alienation occurs so often is not obvious.

The inaccurate information that relatives seem to accumulate certainly plays a role, but the compelling force driving most relatives away from the person with epilepsy is the fear that they will be obliged to help if a seizure occurs. It is upsetting enough to observe a seizure without having the added concern that the health or life of a loved one may depend upon timely action. Most people do not know what to do if a seizure occurs and do not want to be in a situation where that knowledge might be essential. Nevertheless, they frequently continue to burden the immediate family with useless, disturbing, and inaccurate information.

Who was responsible for the epilepsy may become one of the many issues that divide the family. The often guilt-ridden adult with seizures may find relatives reinforcing his gnawing sense of responsibility for the problem. If a child develops epilepsy, parents may burden him with arguments over which of them was at fault, especially if the epilepsy resulted from some type of trauma, such as an automobile accident or sporting injury. When the cause of the seizure disorder is unknown, the accusations often shift to which side of the family the problem was inherited from. The person with epilepsy may withdraw from the rest of the family in order to get away from these disturbing arguments.

Fear and Denial

Relatives of a person with epilepsy often have an inordinate fear that they themselves will develop the disorder. This concern has some statistical validity, at least for brothers and sisters. For 10 percent of the people who develop epilepsy, at least one sibling has a history of seizure disorders. If someone has had only one seizure, the risk that he will have other seizures is substantially greater if he has a brother or sister with epilepsy: for idiopathic seizures, 35 percent of the people who have one seizure will have another within four months if they have an epileptic brother or sister. This simply means that susceptibility to epilepsy, like susceptibility to allergies and heart disease, is greater in some families than in others. The sister of a child with idiopathic seizures will not necessarily develop epilepsy, but the probability that she will have seizures at some time in her life is slightly greater than that of children in the general population.

Children who witness seizures in a sibling may be terrified into paralysis. Paula developed seizures when she was 14 years old. Although she started taking antiepileptic drugs shortly after her first grand mal attack, she continued to have seizures about once a month. Her brother Robert, 3 years younger, did not witness a convulsion until he was 12 years old. He and Paula were helping their father with household chores when Paula abruptly fell to the floor and began to convulse. The father asked Robert to get some pillows to put around Paula to keep her from hurting herself. Obviously terrified, Robert ran into his own room and lay in his bed trembling. Several minutes after his sister had recovered, he emerged from his room in tears. "I wanted to help" was all he could say.

Such paralysis occurs in adults as well. When one young man had a seizure in the presence of his mother-in-law and sister-in-law, they started screaming and abandoned him in terror without even volunteering to get help. The wife of a young man with complex partial seizures recalled with irritation that her husband's sister waited out in the hallway at the hospital when he started to have a seizure. The sister's inability to physically help during this incident was less irritating to the wife than her refusal to stay near enough to provide emotional support.

Family members often refuse to hear that the person has epilepsy. Nathan, who developed epilepsy after an automobile accident, made several attempts to tell his only brother that he had a seizure disorder, and with each attempt his brother turned the discussion to the weather, sports, or another irrelevant matter. His brother did not visit him in the hospital when a bout of frequent seizures obliged Nathan to be admitted, and other relatives provided no comfort or aid to his family when his seizures were at their worst. Nathan could explain such callous behavior only by assuming, "They cannot conceive that I have a problem."

Fault-Finding and Resentment

One of the more pernicious roles played by an unhelpful family is making those closest to the person with seizures feel that they are not doing enough or that they are doing something wrong. The parents, spouses, and siblings of people with epilepsy all face a barrage of irrelevant and largely inaccurate information brought to them under the guise of helpfulness. To avoid this type of harassment, they may disavow all responsibility for control of the seizure disorder, placing it with another family member or the epileptic person himself. This response contributes to the isolation of the person with epilepsy.

Some siblings act as if the disorder is contrived or self-serving. A watchman, who was injured in a robbery attempt and experienced as many as ten seizures a day after undergoing brain surgery, was vexed by his sister's recurrent jibes that he was doing very nicely on his disability income. As a gift at one of the family's celebrations, she bought him a T-shirt that announced that he was a welfare recipient. By minimizing the epileptic person's problems, the family denies him the option of counting on them to offer help or emotional support. Although a small segment of the population with epilepsy does exploit their disability, the belief that people with this type of chronic disorder routinely take unfair advantage of disability insurance is not supported by the facts.

Sometimes brothers, sisters, and other members of the family react as if the epileptic person purposely has the neurologic problem to upset them. Implicit in this reaction is the feeling that the person with seizures is at least partly responsible for his problem. Jena, a young mother whose son temporarily lost consciousness after a head injury, was terrified that the boy might have the seizure disorder her own brother had developed in childhood. She described her brother as generally incompetent and careless. That he had epilepsy and that he had failed to achieve any social goals considered significant by his family were intimately tied together in Jena's view of him. She had little to do with him, largely because she considered him responsible for his poor seizure control. As she saw it, he had not taken charge of his life.

This is not an unusual view for the family to take of the person with epilepsy, and it is often accurate. But this perception ignores the special obligations faced by the person with seizures. People unburdened by epilepsy are not obliged to constantly monitor their own behavior and take medication. What the family often sees is someone living in the careless manner in which most people live, but suffering special consequences.

When a child has epilepsy, it is important to give the non-epileptic siblings their share of parental attention and to recognize their limitations. They should not be required to help manage the epileptic child's seizures or to provide emotional support for their parents. The epileptic child's brothers and sisters face their own problems and have a right to the same help that parents give the child with epilepsy.

When an adult has epilepsy, the friction in the immediate and extended family must be minimized, and some of the burden of achieving this invariably falls upon the person with the seizures. Much of what seems like malice or insensitivity in family members is nothing more than denial of a frightening condition, the epilepsy. Relatives who do not have the problem cannot truly understand what the person with epilepsy must face every day, and they should not be expected to understand. By ignoring what could easily be taken as abrasive remarks and behavior, the person with epilepsy may be able to preserve family relationships that will prove invaluable over a lifetime.

Chapter Nine

Personality Changes and Violence

What happens to the thoughts, behavior, personality, and mood of people with epilepsy has been disputed for decades. Some physicians have insisted that none of these brain functions is altered by seizures, and others have claimed that specific defects may appear in people with specific types of seizures. The controversy is far from settled.

What may be said with some confidence is that many people exhibit no change in thoughts, feelings, or actions as a direct result of their seizure disorder but that many others do have psychologic changes associated with particular types of seizures. This does not necessarily mean that the psychologic changes are caused by the epilepsy itself. These changes and the seizure disorder may simply be two manifestations of one nervous system disease or injury.

Problems with mood and behavior develop in people with epilepsy at least as often as in people with other chronic diseases. Depression and anger are appropriate and unavoidable when the seizure disorder is poorly controlled or when treatment measures are causing problems of their own. However, some people with epilepsy exhibit more disruptive behavior than can be attributed to depression. Some of this behavior is undeniably violent and may have tragically damaging consequences. Violent behavior may occur during the ictus of the seizure, but most of it happens during postictal confusion. There remains, however, in a small segment of the population with epilepsy, much peculiar and some truly sociopathic behavior that is unrelated to specific seizures.

Opinions differ widely about the relationship among these personality changes, violent behavior, and particular seizure disorders, but the consensus is that purposefully violent behavior is not characteristic of any type of epilepsy. Aggressive, destructive behavior during a seizure has been clearly documented in very few instances. People with epilepsy certainly may damage property or injure people who try to subdue them while they are confused or convulsing, but this type of destructiveness is obviously not intentional. After the seizure proper, the victim may still be too confused to act coherently for several minutes or even hours and may cause what appears to be much more intentional damage. This is not the most common type of behavior in the postictal period, a period during which most people are lethargic and confused, but neither is it extremely rare.

Personality Traits

Fewer than 25 percent of people with seizure disorders are free of any cognitive, behavioral, or simply neurologic problems, and about 50 percent have significant psychological or social problems that show up in their daily activities and behavior. Although depression, excessive anxiety, self-denigration, hypochondria, confused thinking, excessive sensitivity, and a pervasive dissatisfaction are commonly reported by and observed in adults with epilepsy, an epileptic person is most likely to have only some or none of these traits. Not surprisingly, many people with epilepsy are embarrassed when their seizures occur, feel considerable resentment that they have this problem at all, feel that their worth is diminished because of the disorder, and feel less accepted by others because of their condition. These are not abnormal personality traits in any sense, and in fact 70 percent of those with epilepsy feel neither unreasonably limited nor subject to special treatment because of their seizures; but when these feelings are persistent, they do interfere with normal activities.

Unquestionable psychologic impairment is most common in people with complex partial seizures, especially in those whose seizures first appear during adolescence. Developing epilepsy before or after adolescence results in a lower overall rate of personality disorders, an observation that is not explained by current notions on the evolution of seizures. This phenomenon may occur because of a special vulnerability in adolescence to problems that interfere with the development of a stable self-image.

Although substantial psychologic problems in people with idiopathic seizures are fairly uncommon, some people with complex partial seizures have problems ranging from hyperactive behavior and violence to sexual dysfunction and hypochondria. Schizophrenia and psychotic depressions are rare in people with epilepsy, but they appear more frequently in people with complex partial seizures than in those with any other type of epilepsy. This observation reinforces the impression that people with seizures originating in damaged structures in the temporal lobe are particularly vulnerable to psychiatric disorders.

Obsessive and paranoid traits are especially characteristic of people whose seizures originate in the temporal lobe and develop before puberty. The paranoid ideas these people have are often religious or mystical in character. Some have multiple religious conversions after mystical experiences. God speaks to them directly and tells them what religion to practice and preach. In addition to having this feeling of divine importance or a religious mission, these people often ascribe great significance to commonplace events. If a book accidentally falls open, a passage on the page may be seen as a warning or a prophecy. A fellow worker's cough may be interpreted as a criticism. Inconsequential events may be recorded in detailed diaries as part of a compulsion to write down everything.

In many instances, the personality changes that may occur when someone develops epilepsy are neither peculiar nor undesirable. A family may notice that a previously abusive member has mellowed with the evolution of the seizure disorder. An embarrassingly reserved member of the family may become more outgoing. These kinds of changes in personality obviously do not require treatment. When a serious personality disorder develops, however, and when treatment of the seizures alone does not correct it, psychiatric intervention may be necessary.

Mood Disturbances

Depression and other mood disturbances experienced by some people with epilepsy are more than just emotional reactions to uncontrollable seizures. The incidence of serious depressions in people with epilepsy has remained largely unchanged over the past thirty years despite substantial advances in seizure control. Serious mood disturbances are not limited to people who require hospitalization for frequent seizures or other neurologic problems; 17 to 25 percent of people with epilepsy who are not hospitalized have psychologic problems that interfere with their daily functioning, and at least 10 percent need psychiatric intervention or hospitalization at some time in their lives.

A suicide attempt often brings the patient to the attention of psychiatrists. This self-destructive bent is not just a response to chronic disability, since people with epilepsy who have the most severe mood disturbances are often much less disabled than people with other chronic medical problems who exhibit no mood disorders. The severity of the mood disorder does not parallel the severity of the seizure disorder.

Whether a mood disturbance is independent of the epilepsy or simply another facet of the seizure disorder is not always obvious. Some people, especially those whose seizures originate in the temporal lobe, develop overwhelming fear with the seizures or between seizure episodes. When it is part of the seizure proper (the ictus), this is usually called ictal fear. It is the most common emotion felt during seizures, and it is experienced by as many as 22 percent of those whose seizures originate in the temporal lobe. The evaluation of this baseless emotion is complicated by the appearance of a more abiding fear in many of these people, a fear that lasts for hours or days between the obvious seizure episodes.

Treating mood disturbances with antidepressant drugs poses special problems for people with epilepsy. Many antidepressants, such as the tricyclic compounds imipramine (Tofranil) and amitriptyline (Elavil), lower the seizure threshold and may be particularly dangerous for depressed people who might ignore instructions on how to take the medication.

To treat severe depression in people without seizure disorders, the physician has the option of using electroconvulsive therapy. In epileptic people, however, this is even more dangerous than antidepressants, because shock treatment is nothing more than an induced seizure. Both pharmaceutical and electroshock approaches to the depression carry the risk of exacerbating the seizure disorder.

This does not mean that the depression, anxiety, or fear experienced by people with epilepsy should not be treated; what it means is that drugs or electroconvulsive therapy must be applied with constant attention to the increased risk of seizures. To leave these severe mood disturbances untreated is to run the risk of suicide.

Violent Behavior

The damage done by an epileptic person during and shortly after a seizure is random and gives the person neither personal gain nor satisfaction. In fact, much of the damage may be inflicted upon items the person specifically tries to protect. A vase pushed out of the way in the last confused moment before a generalized convulsion may be broken; a child inadvertently placed on a precarious support during the altered perceptions of a partial seizure may be injured. Inadvertent destructiveness is most common in the postictal period.

Deciding whether the damage is intentional is also most difficult during the postictal period. The person may seem fully alert and aware of what he is doing and may make threats that seem too well-conceived to be the ranting of a confused mind. Even the amnesia or imperfect recall of events during this violent period is difficult for witnesses to believe, partly because there is a seamless transition from the confusion and irritability of the postictal period to the clarity and remorse of the interictal period.

It is understandable that onlookers think the disorganized aggressiveness results from malicious intent, but in fact the damage is done because of confusion rather than malice or anger. The anger may appear authentic, but the justifications for it are illogical or delusional. Perhaps an analogy for the person's state of mind during this period is dreamlike; in dreams, things are said and done out of confusion that would never happen normally. People who can remember even fragments of the seizure after it is over are almost always embarrassed and remorseful.

Violent behavior during a seizure is occasionally a reaction to well-formed delusions or hallucinations, which may result from a tumor or other physical problem in the brain (Figure 6). People may react to their threatening hallucinations with outbursts directed toward real people around them. A cup of coffee in someone's hand may be seen as a gun. A casual greeting may be heard as an angry threat. The victim of the seizure reacts to these menacing delusions with terror or violence. This ictal violence can be more dangerous than the postictal confusion and irritability that account for most aggressive behavior in people with epilepsy, but the violence is too random and too disorganized to cause much real injury to anyone except the person with seizures himself.

The belief that criminal activities can be the result of epileptic seizures has been reinforced by the increasing number of pleas in criminal court alleging that a defendant accused of an aggressive, violent, or simply felonious act was having a seizure at the time. The argument is that the defendant cannot be held responsible for the crime because when the crime was committed he was suffering from altered consciousness imposed by the epilepsy. Complex partial seizures are the seizure

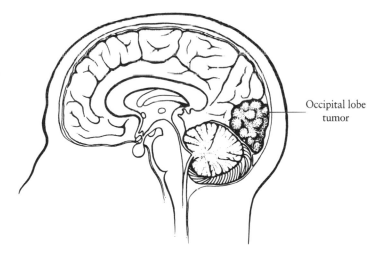

Occipital lobe
tumor

FIGURE 6. Tumor overlying the brain. A person with hallucinations may have a psychiatric problem, but occasionally hallucinations are caused by structural lesions in or on the brain. A tumor pressing on the occipital lobe can cause focal sensory seizures that are mistaken for delusions or hallucinations.

disorder most often invoked as the basis for the altered mental state, but most neurologists do not believe that repeated violence and destructive behavior can be ascribed to this or any seizure type. People with epilepsy may commit robbery, assault, rape, or murder, but not because they have epilepsy. They commit crimes for the same reasons that people without epilepsy commit crimes. Criminal intent does not develop from the epilepsy.

Relationship of Violence to Seizure Type

Many studies have suggested that violence associated with epilepsy is most likely to occur if the victim of the seizure disorder has complex partial seizures arising in the temporal lobe of the brain, but the findings in this area have been very inconsistent. There clearly are many people in epilepsy clinics with seizures arising from temporal lobe damage who have obvious mental illness, peculiar social behavior, or unusual personality traits. A few of these people have frank psychoses, some have personality disorders that keep them from developing relationships or being gainfully employed, and some exhibit clearly violent or destructive behavior. But these people are quite atypical of people with epilepsy. They are usually indigent, have poor seizure control, and exhibit numerous social problems. Highly compliant, socially integrated people with well-controlled epilepsy are less likely to be in the clinic group; they do not require regular supervision.

Studies that have linked complex partial seizures with aggressive, destructive, or otherwise sociopathic behavior have been primarily preoperative or postoperative evaluations of people with intractable seizures treated surgically. In these people, definite structural damage to the temporal lobe is found in 80 percent of cases, a relatively high rate of pathology for a population with epilepsy. Aggressive behavior, manifested by unpredictable outbursts of anger during the interictal period, is the most common psychologic problem described. Still, the current consensus leans away from any clear association between damage to the temporal lobe and violent behavior. Even those studies that do suggest a causal relationship between temporal lobe seizures and aggression in some people recognize that most people with this type of seizure disorder are not unusually aggressive. Male sex, low IQ, lack of religious ties, and juvenile behavior problems are all more important factors than epilepsy in the appearance of violent or destructive behavior disorders in people with epilepsy. There is little consistent evidence that criminal behavior occurs more often in victims of complex partial seizures than in people with grand mal seizures or, for that matter, in the general population.

Some studies have suggested that the people with epilepsy most likely to show irrational destructive or abusive behavior as adults are those whose seizures start early in childhood. When the anterior temporal lobe is surgically removed, the aggressive behavior disappears for more than six years in 20 percent of the people so treated. But whether a person's age at the onset of the seizure disorder is important in the development of aggressive behavior is still controversial. Of the people with epilepsy who do exhibit aggressive behavior, 41 percent have a history of permanent separation from one or both parents before the age of 15. For many of these people, disruptive behavior at an early age, rather than seizures, initially brings them to medical attention.

A complicating factor is that much of what is interpreted as psychopathology may be fairly routine postictal signs of a neurological disturbance. People whose seizures originate in the temporal lobes may have problems with word-finding during the interictal period. Presumably this is nothing more than a sign of disturbed temporal lobe function persisting long after obvious seizures have abated. Much of the peculiar behavior attributed to people with temporal lobe seizures may be caused by similar interictal disturbances.

In general, children with temporal lobe seizures alone do

not have unprovoked attacks of rage. In some cases episodes of rage and hyperactive behavior occur when the seizures first develop, but they become less frequent as the child matures. Recurrent depression becomes more of a problem in adulthood. Some adults with complex partial epilepsy are remarkably irritable and have profound mood swings.

John developed complex partial seizures when he was 45 years old. Before the disorder appeared he was always even-tempered and never raised his voice, used obscenities, or exhibited any violent behavior. "If the ceiling fell down next to him," his wife said, "he'd simply get up and move his chair." But as his seizures progressed from minor changes in consciousness to long spells of confusion with peculiar gestures and a tendency to wander, violent outbursts became routine. When some teenagers did not move out of his way as he was trying to park, he raced his car toward them, shouting obscenities at them as they jumped aside. When a woman tried to push ahead of him at a supermarket, he picked up her groceries and flung them to the ground. When his family questioned him about his violent behavior, he denied it and became abusive toward them. The abusiveness never occurred during a seizure or during the postictal period, but his wife noticed that his most violent episodes would be followed within hours by a seizure.

What may be most important in determining whether a person with complex partial seizures has violent outbursts is the type of damage that has occurred in the temporal lobe, rather than the type of seizure exhibited. The abnormal personality traits, changes in personality, and seizures may all be separate manifestations of a problem in the brain, rather than being causally related to one another.

Comparing episodes of violent behavior in people with complex partial seizures and those with generalized seizures, some investigators find no relationship between the incidence of aggression and the seizure type. In those with generalized seizures, people who are younger or who have myoclonic seizures are less likely to be violent than older people with tonic-clonic seizures. People with akinetic seizures, a type of generalized seizure in which the affected person temporarily stops all movement except breathing, have a clearly increased incidence of violent behavior. What does occur frequently in adults with complex partial seizures is episodic abusiveness to family members. This is occasionally manifest as wife beating or husband beating. These violent outbursts are unrelated to apparent seizure episodes but may be related to the overall level of seizure control.

Episodic Dyscontrol

Concern that aggressive criminal behavior might result from injuries to particular parts of the brain has prompted considerable study of aggression and violence after brain damage. The results of these studies, as well as the procedures used, are controversial. One problem is that often aggressive populations are studied to determine whether they show an unusually high incidence of epilepsy. A better method would be to start with a population of people known to have seizures and then to determine if this group shows an excess of destructive behavior.

Even though some studies of prison populations have suggested that epilepsy is common in sociopaths, the prisoners usually studied have questionable evidence of seizures. More objective studies do not support the notion that epilepsy is highly correlated with criminal behavior. According to fairly reliable studies from England, the prevalence of epilepsy is only slightly greater in prison populations than in the general population and is associated with other contributing factors such as a history of head injuries.

Research on violent individuals and criminal populations has fostered the notion that a disorganized emotional or mental state is involved in many violent acts. This has been called the episodic dyscontrol syndrome. People with this syndrome have discrete bouts of violent behavior that last minutes or hours. These paroxysms are largely unprovoked and are occasionally preceded by abnormal sensations. After an episode the person often complains of headache or drowsiness. Implicit in the grouping of these behavior disorders into a syndrome is that a common nervous system disorder, perhaps an epileptic disorder, underlies the violence.

People with episodic dyscontrol share several characteristics besides their violent behavior. They are usually men who come from poor families, have little formal education, and exhibit sociopathic behavior by their twenties or early thirties. Their fathers often are chronic alcoholics and child abusers. More than 70 percent of those who develop episodic dyscontrol as adults are hyperactive in childhood, and half claim to have had staring spells, unrelated to violent behavior, that lasted seconds and involved "altered consciousness." These people are very remorseful, and about 50 percent claim that they have tried to kill themselves. Alcohol increases the frequency and severity of their criminal outbursts. More than 30 percent admit to sexual problems, including impotence, transvestitism, and obsessive abstinence from sex.

An episode of uncontrolled violence may be preceded by visual illusions, altered hearing, nausea, or pins-and-needles sensations. After the attack, some people claim that they do not remember what happened. Those that recall it deny that they could control it. Actually, these claims are fairly common for people accused of committing crimes: 72 percent of juveniles accused of committing violent crimes claim memory lapses, blackouts, dizziness, and dreamlike states during the crime and fatigue after the crime. These phenomena are probably subjective changes associated with excitement, rather than with epilepsy. On the assumption that epilepsy might be playing a role in these violent outbursts, some people with episodic dyscontrol have been treated with antiepileptic drugs. Sixty-eight percent reported some improvement while on phenytoin. This is probably not significant, since the syndrome usually disappears on its own as the person gets older. Episodic dyscontrol rarely appears in anyone over 50 years of age.

Any objective study of violent populations is further complicated by what these people have to gain if they can convince a court of law that their underlying problem is epilepsy. Studies that show an incidence of epilepsy in prison populations ten times as high as in the general population are misleading. Given the curious acceptance of epilepsy as a cause of violent behavior, a defense based on a nervous system disorder is likely to be offered in court. Unfortunately, the diagnosis of epilepsy in most cases relies heavily on the person's own testimony, and so an excessive number of epileptic cases are discovered during trials. Many of these accused people admit that alcohol or other drugs played a role in their destructive behavior, and this too argues against their having epilepsy.

Evidence that epilepsy is an important or constant element in this episodic dyscontrol syndrome is weak. The syndrome is probably a somewhat consistent personality disorder appearing in criminals, regardless of whether or not they also have a seizure disorder. One reason the term episodic dyscontrol syndrome has had some popularity is that it does not label this behavior disorder as epilepsy.

Fugue States

In some types of seizures, the person may enter a protracted trancelike state. This is an extremely rare situation, but it does occur with generalized absence (petit mal) and complex partial (psychomotor) seizures. This is called a fugue state, a term more commonly used to refer to episodes of wandering seen in people with schizophrenia or other psychoses. People with fugue states caused by epilepsy may be much less mobile and self-sufficient than people with schizophrenic episodes, and their protracted episodes of confusion are also called twilight states if they appear to be part of the postictal period.

During the epileptic fugue state, an electroencephalogram will reveal diffuse electrical changes characteristic of seizures, making this a form of status epilepticus (see Chapter 10). After the episode the person will generally not remember what happened. During the fugue or twilight state the person will not be able to perform complex activities. When those people travel, they get lost. If they are not given shelter, they stay exposed. In fugue and twilight states it is remarkable that the person is conscious and active at all. Their activities usually do not appear normal. Someone encountering a person in this condition would suspect that something is profoundly wrong. Amnesia is a relatively minor aspect of the fugue or twilight state.

Domestic Abuse

When violent behavior does occur in a person with epilepsy, family members are often the targets. Family members are usually injured because they attempt to deal with the person having seizures as if he were perfectly rational and coherent. The wife, husband, or child trying hardest to cope with the epileptic person's erratic behavior is at the greatest risk.

Although most abusiveness in people with epilepsy is clearly a part of the seizures themselves, some people exhibit abusive behavior that seems unconnected to seizures. When the abusiveness is largely unprovoked, lack of seizure control should be considered, and suppression of the seizures should be the first objective of treatment.

Abusive behavior need not occur during the seizure to be clearly related to it. One wife noticed that her husband would go through three typical stages before a seizure. He would become depressed, then increasingly irritable and verbally abusive, and then he would develop unequivocal seizures. In his irritable stage he repeatedly interfered with his wife's attempts to get medical help for him. This man did not physically abuse his wife, but another man with a similar pattern of progressive irritability consulted physicians specifically because he was beating his wife. After their seizures, both men were remorseful, but their wives doubted their sincerity and were afraid of them. For both men, improved seizure control resulted in less violent behavior. But the best way to decrease a person's violence varies with specific features of each person's disorder.

When a husband, wife, child, or parent becomes threatening and abusive, family members should assume that the episode is irrational and potentially dangerous. Whether this outburst occurs during the ictus of a seizure, in the postictal period, or between seizures, direct confrontation with the violent person should be avoided. Trying to restrain a violent person during the postictal period risks substantial injury to both the person with epilepsy and the would-be helper. If an epileptic person becomes violent when a seizure has not occurred, family members should take this as a signal to keep their contact with that person to a minimum.

For any person who shows a tendency to violent behavior, firearms should be made inaccessible. Many family members believe they must stay nearby during the violent episodes as a sign of their trust. This type of behavior ignores the seizure victim's impaired condition and invites tragedy.

If the person's violent episodes endanger himself and if family members might be injured in trying to protect him, the family should seek outside assistance. If the degree of confusion and potential for injury is relatively slight, an emergency ambulance crew or other paramedical professionals should be able to manage the situation. If the violence is more substantial, police intervention may be necessary. The family's first responsibility is to avoid tragedy, not to avoid embarrassment or hurt feelings.

Violence with Improved Seizure Control

With some seizure disorders, such as complex partial seizures, the person may show increasingly violent behavior as the seizures are better controlled. Richard, a 40-year-old man with poorly controlled seizures, was started on carbamazepine after having seizures more than once a month for several years. With this medication his seizures recurred much less often, but he found himself flying into rages. He broke furniture and beat his wife. She was terrified by Richard's abrupt change in behavior and sought additional medical help. Rather than allowing him to have seizures and become more subdued, the physician increased the antiepileptic medications to make him completely seizure-free and added antidepressant medication. With this change in drugs, Richard became less depressed, less violent, and free of seizures, but his wife was still afraid of him. Whenever Richard looked irritable, she would try to avoid his company. Although his violence had been transient, it caused a lasting rift in their marriage.

For many people with complex partial seizures and violent outbursts, the outbursts seem to follow long seizure-free intervals. The abusive behavior lasts hours to days and may end abruptly when a seizure occurs. During this irritable period, the person resists all efforts to calm him and broods over imagined slights or insults. Serious injury to others is unlikely, and when the anger abates the person is usually remorseful and apologetic. He remembers how he behaved and may promise to avoid such behavior in the future. Of course, the promise will be forgotten when the next imagined slight provokes another episode of anger.

When control of a seizure disorder increases the frequency of violent episodes between seizures, some physicians allow their patients' seizures to remain incompletely controlled. Allowing recurrent seizures is risky, however, because injury to the person or status epilepticus may result. Combining treatment of the seizures with antidepressant medications is a safer approach; this should generally be undertaken with the assistance of a psychiatrist who has expertise in treating patients with neurologic disorders.

It is worth noting that much of the violence observed in people whose seizures originate in the temporal lobes abates after surgery. This fact has been offered as a justification for using temporal lobe surgery to deal with violent behavior itself. But the long-term effects of the surgery are controversial, and the cause of the observed changes is poorly understood. This type of surgery cannot be considered as a way of managing violent behavior (see Chapter 11).

Suicide Attempts

Self-destructive behavior is common in people with epilepsy. It may range from inappropriate risk-taking to unequivocal suicide attempts. Depression often accompanies any chronic health problem such as heart disease or multiple sclerosis, but in some types of epilepsy the disorder itself probably contributes to the mood disturbance that leads to self-destructive behavior. People with seizure disorders have ready access to dangerous medications, and, sadly, many of them use those drugs to attempt suicide.

Sometimes these drugs can contribute to a lethal outcome even if the person does not intend to commit suicide. For example, driving a car when seizure control is poor is dangerous under the best of circumstances, but especially so when dosages of antiepileptic drugs have recently been changed, because the change in medication may slow the person's reaction times.

Attempted suicide is common among people with all types of seizures. Along with lethal events that are a direct expression of the disorder, such as untreated status epilepticus and seizure-related accidents, suicide ranks as a leading cause of death in people with epilepsy. As in any population of people, there is also a group whose cause of death appears to be accidental or is never described as anything more than an unexplained cardiac arrest. The high incidence of accidental and unexplained deaths in the population with seizures suggests that the true incidence of suicide may be even higher than has been documented.

Some studies attribute 12 to 20 percent of deaths in people with epilepsy to suicide—five times the rate of attempted suicide in the general population (which is 32.5 per thousand). The rate of suicide attempts among those with complex partial seizures may be as much as 25 times greater than that of the general population.

Two factors place people with epilepsy at special risk: they have a high incidence of depressive illnesses, and they have easy access to nonviolent instruments of suicide, namely antiepileptic drugs. Of those with epilepsy who attempt suicide, 84 percent try to poison or overdose themselves, and 65 percent use antiepileptics.

About two thirds of those who attempt suicide by self-poisoning take an antiepileptic they have been prescribed, and another 15 percent combine antiepileptics with other drugs. Overdoses of phenobarbital have always been especially common among people attempting suicide; the respiratory depressant action of phenobarbital is often purposely enhanced by alcohol. Even though phenobarbital is being supplanted by other antiepileptics, some of the antiepileptic medications in use are metabolized to phenobarbital, and others can depress breathing even though they are not barbiturates. When medication is closely supervised, the suicide rate is lower: people in hospitals or other institutions are much less likely to commit suicide than are people with epilepsy outside such facilities.

Men with epilepsy are more likely to attempt suicide than women, and both are more inclined to make serious suicide attempts when they are unemployed. Sixty percent of those with seizure disorders who attempt suicide are under 30 years of age. Repeated attempts are twice as common in people with epilepsy as in people without epilepsy: 74 percent of people with seizures who fail in a suicide attempt will try again. Obviously the person at greatest risk of repeated suicide attempts is the one who fails through misinformation alone. A person who takes a massive dose of phenytoin and suffers little more than difficulty in walking, blurred vision, nausea, and vomiting may try again with a more effective drug. Careful observation and aggressive treatment of such people are important in any plan to avert suicide.

Major psychiatric disorders, such as schizophrenia and manic-depressive (bipolar) psychoses, are no more common in suicidal populations with epilepsy than in suicidal populations without it, but there is a higher incidence of personality disorders in suicidal people with epilepsy. Epileptic people face special social problems because of their chronic disorder, and sometimes they have the added disadvantage of personality disorders that limit their ability to cope with their unusual burdens. All this contributes to frustration and anger that may make the person self-destructive.

To reduce the risk of additional suicide attempts, the family and physician must consider the events leading to the initial self-destructive action. Multiple problems usually contribute to the person's feeling of hopelessness, but there is often a distressing incident or an unresolvable problem that triggers the final dramatic gesture or sincere attempt at self-destruction. Some people fall into despair out of profound guilt over being constantly dependent or sick. One woman with epilepsy tried to kill herself because she felt responsible for her daughter's seizures. Problems with seizure control or difficulty in keeping a job are often given as reasons for suicide attempts, but the true reasons may be more subtle. For example, conflict with a spouse over financial worries or problems with seizure control may be more important in precipitating a suicide attempt than the unemployment or the seizures themselves.

Self-Destructive Behavior through Noncompliance

A person's decision to stop taking antiepileptics may bring on the sometimes lethal convulsive disorder called status epilepticus. Although such potentially dangerous behavior as refusing medication is generally not included in statistics on suicide, it probably accounts for as much injury and death as do outright suicide attempts. A person with epilepsy can inflict considerable self-damage with minimal effort and planning.

Equally dangerous is a refusal to comply with restrictions on activity. Swimming, driving a car, rock climbing, and commuting by subway can all pose substantial threats to a person whose seizures are poorly controlled. Men especially resist giving up these prerogatives, which seem to be tied to their self-images. One man with epilepsy foolishly insisted on driving when his family took trips even though others in the car could drive. He explained this as a way of testing himself, and members of his family did not actively resist. Ironically, when the safety of his entire family was not threatened, he rarely insisted on driving. He seemed to cling to his role as head of the family more than to his own image of himself as a driver.

Minimizing Risks

To avoid tragedy, the epileptic person and the family must recognize that the risk of self-injury exists. Allowing a family member with poorly controlled seizures to drive a car while the family is in it is a denial of risk that can be lethal for the entire family. Most states allow people with epilepsy to drive if they have been seizure-free for 6 to 12 months, whether or not they require medication. This is a reasonable position for the family to adopt in dealing with a member with seizures who is inclined to disregard the law.

When people with epilepsy are depressed, nothing is gained by leaving them to "work it out on their own." Problems, conflicts, and concerns should be explored with a psychotherapist or a physician familiar with the person's illness and life circumstances. Self-destructive behavior, and even talk about suicide, should not be ignored. Anything resembling a suicide attempt should immediately be brought to the attention of a physician. Depression can be effectively treated, and the risks of self-destructive behavior can be minimized, but only if the problem is managed energetically and intelligently by experienced professionals. A suicide attempt is not something to be dealt with by sympathetic remarks over the dinner table. A therapist or physician should be involved immediately in treating the depression.

Chapter Ten

Diagnosing Epilepsy

Before epilepsy can be properly treated, the seizure disorder must be recognized. A generalized tonic-clonic seizure is obvious after only one attack, but other disorders may not be suspected for weeks or months. The infant who has a generalized tonic-clonic seizure with a high fever will be quickly brought to a physician by the horrified parents, but parents of another child may observe several dozen staring spells or drop attacks without suspecting a medical problem. If they do not perceive the problem for some time, the gaps in the child's consciousness may interfere with learning, and the child may even be mistakenly diagnosed as mentally retarded.

If bedwetting is the only symptom of generalized seizures in an adult, the person may conceal the problem for years before mentioning it to a physician, and even then the physician may investigate the symptom only from a urological—rather than a neurological—standpoint. Older adults with bedwetting in their sleep are often considered prematurely senile; epilepsy is suspected by neither the elderly person nor the family. An

TABLE 22
Causes of Epilepsy in Adults

Idiopathic (unknown)
Trauma
Infection
Stroke
Hemorrhage
Tumor
Vascular malformation
Vascular inflammation
Parasites
Poisons
Drugs

older person who loses consciousness during the day may be misconstrued as having had a stroke, which some people incorrectly believe to be a reasonable consequence of senility. This misinterpretation of increasing seizure activity leaves the person at considerable risk of being injured by the seizure disorder itself. Even when a lapse in consciousness causes a fall, producing a head injury, the fall is often interpreted as the reason for the person's subsequent confusion, and epilepsy is not suspected.

Of course, not all alterations of consciousness are the result of seizures. Any person who is thought to have seizures should be investigated for other explanations as well (see Table 22). In the elderly, heart problems, such as subtle irregularities in the heartbeat, can profoundly affect the flow of blood to the brain and produce transient unconsciousness. A Holter monitor recording of cardiac activity over the course of 24 hours or more may be needed to detect the irregular rhythm. A routine electrocardiogram (EKG) will reveal structural damage to the heart muscle, disturbances of conduction between different chambers of the heart, or persistent irregularities of heartbeat.

Younger people may have metabolic or anatomical problems that cause fainting. In some, coughing or urinating will trigger an exaggerated vascular reflex and induce fainting. Hyperventilation—an aberrant breathing pattern that commonly develops with acute anxiety—may also produce fainting and may be mistaken for a seizure disorder. Despite its popularity as a diagnosis, transient hypoglycemia (low blood sugar) rarely is responsible for fainting in people who are not taking medication to lower their blood sugar.

History and Exam

After the affected person or family member recognizes a possible seizure disorder and brings it to the attention of a physician, the physician will attempt to establish the cause, or at least eliminate all treatable causes. With epilepsy, as with any medical complaint, the first step in the physician's investigation is to take a medical history. This includes accounts by the patient, her family, and other witnesses of what happened during the seizure, during the days and weeks around the time of the seizure, and during other illnesses she may have had.

Unfortunately, an accurate history is difficult to obtain in the case of seizures. The patient is often unaware of what occurred during the seizure and may have a confused and incomplete memory of events immediately preceding and following it. Family and friends are usually better sources for descriptions of the events surrounding the seizure, but they may have been too upset to remember exactly what happened. Since treatment is dictated by the type of seizure, and since the type of seizure is established largely by the description of seizure characteristics, every attempt should be made to give the physician a complete and accurate picture of the seizure.

To complicate matters, many patients deliberately conceal information relevant to their disorder. A person may be too embarrassed to report bedwetting, and the family may fail to mention personality changes for fear of angering or offending the patient. If the seizures have evolved from fainting attacks to generalized convulsions, the patient and the family may cling to an early diagnosis of hypoglycemia or hardening of the arteries and not fully discuss the changing pattern of the attacks.

Obviously, the evaluation of any person with episodes suggestive of altered consciousness, transient involuntary movements, or fleeting sensory phenomena must include a series of questions that clarify what the person has been experiencing. The physician will ask both the patient and family members about urinary and fecal incontinence, aimless violence, personality changes, and sexual dysfunction. Most of the details of what happens during the seizure itself can be described only by witnesses, since the patient is not conscious, though patients may sometimes recall paralysis, panic, or other abnormal phenomena.

Drug and alcohol use and abuse, including illegal drugs, should be discussed honestly. Cocaine, amphetamines, and other widely used recreational drugs may cause seizures, as may many prescription drugs (see Table 23). How much and in what form the person consumes alcohol must also be clarified, since seizures can occur during acute alcohol withdrawal. The patient and family members should try to answer all of these questions forthrightly, without taking offense. Physicians know that many well-educated people abuse drugs and alcohol as often as the poorly educated; they cannot assume that well-groomed, articulate, urbane, and financially successful people are not drug- or alcohol-dependent.

A complete physical examination is basic to the investigation of every person suspected of having a seizure disorder.

TABLE 23

Drug Use Associated with Seizures

Seizures with use	Seizures with withdrawal
Cocaine	Barbiturates
Amphetamines	Alcohol
Methaqualone	Benzodiazepines
Aminophylline	Phencyclidine

Special attention to the nervous system is appropriate, but careful observation of all other major body systems is also important. Large brown spots over several areas of the skin may indicate neurofibromatosis, a hereditary disorder that can cause brain tumors. Minor joint changes may be the first indication of systemic lupus erythematosus (SLE), a vascular disease that can cause transient brain dysfunction. A complete physical examination will also help to exclude problems that imitate seizures. An irregular pulse may be the first indication of an unsuspected cardiac arrhythmia. A heart murmur may prompt investigations that reveal diseased heart valves; if blood clots periodically break off the diseased valves and go to the brain, they can clog vital arteries and provoke fainting spells. In a child, odd movements of the arms, shoulders, or face and sniffing, snorting, or smacking sounds may turn out to be a tic disorder or Tourette syndrome rather than epilepsy.

Electroencephalography

Most useful in the investigation of seizure disorders is the electroencephalograph, a device for amplifying and displaying changes in the electrical activity of the most superficial layers of the brain. Electrodes placed on the scalp detect fluctuations in voltage originating in several different areas of the brain. These fluctuations are amplified by special circuits in the electroencephalograph and are displayed as oscillations of voltage-sensitive needles or as waves and spikes on electronic displays. This record of what are called brain waves is the electroencephalogram (EEG).

In most cases, the EEG will help to diagnose a seizure disorder, and in some cases it can even suggest the underlying cause. Although an abnormal EEG can occur in someone who does not have seizures, it is good evidence that seizures are occurring in a person with poorly understood motor, sensory, or mental symptoms.

Several patterns of brain waves are normal in children and adults. When the person is relaxed and has both eyes closed, rhythmical oscillations in electrical activity arising from the back part of the head will appear with a frequency of about 8 to 12 cycles per second (hertz). This alpha activity, as it is called, disappears when the person opens his eyes or attempts mental tasks such as multiplication or division (see Figure 7). More toward the front of the head, the EEG will consist of irregular combinations of waves at varying frequencies. With drowsiness, the overall frequency of the waves gets slower.

The electroencephalograph displays brain activity as waves, spikes, and electrical silence. A wave that is sharply contoured and lasts less than one-fifth of a second is called a sharp wave. When a sharply contoured wave lasts less than one-twelfth of a second, it is called a spike. Seizure activity usually appears as spikes and slow waves. When they arise from a limited area over the brain, spikes and slow waves generally indicate structural abnormalities in or near that part of the brain (see Figure 8). There are several exceptions to this rule, and being aware of those exceptions keeps the physician from diagnosing brain disorders where they do not exist.

Sharp waves, for example, may be normal at the back of the head in an elderly person. Spikes that appear to be pointing downward and occur at 14 or 6 cycles per second may arise in the temporal regions during sleep in healthy young adults or adolescents, and they do not indicate epilepsy. With arousal from sleep, there may be high-voltage waves with small notches that resemble spikes and slow waves. These are generally seen in childhood and are normal.

All of these variants can lead to considerable misinterpretation of the EEG, especially when a seizure is suspected. Various maneuvers can make abnormal brain activity more apparent. Hyperventilation or sleep may enhance a spike focus that is not prominent when the person is awake or breathing at a

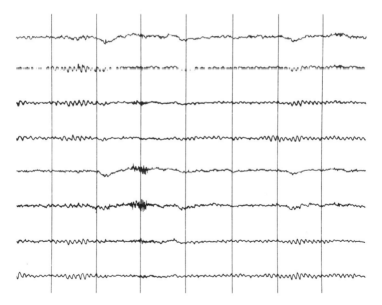

FIGURE 7. Normal electroencephalogram. The vertical lines on this record indicate 1-second intervals. The fourth and eighth horizontal lines most clearly show the small rhythmical waves called alpha waves. This young man had alpha waves with a frequency of 10 per second. The small spikes in the middle of the fifth and sixth horizontal lines are from muscle activity about the head.

normal rate. Flashing lights may elicit spike activity in an otherwise normal EEG.

Although the EEG alone will not firmly establish the cause of a seizure disorder, some patterns limit the possibilities. In children, periodic discharges occurring at a rate of less than one discharge every four seconds often develop with subacute sclerosing panencephalitis, a rare but lethal degenerative disease of the brain. When the discharge rate is greater than once every two seconds, the underlying brain disease may be Creutzfeldt-Jakob disease, a slow-viral illness causing dementia in adults, or Tay-Sachs disease, an inborn error of metabolism causing dementia in children. With brain damage resulting from poisons or anoxia, a more variable periodic pattern occasionally appears in which the sharp waves are much more prominent on one side. This pattern is called periodic lateralized epileptiform discharges (PLEDs), and it may also

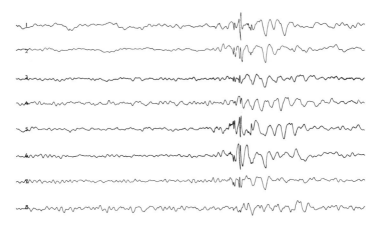

FIGURE 8. Spike-and-slow-wave discharge. Two-thirds of the way across the page there is a high-amplitude spike with associated high-amplitude slow waves. This type of activity often appears between seizures in a person with epilepsy. The areas most involved with the abnormal electrical activity are likely to be the regions of the brain in which the seizure activity is originating.

be produced by tumors, strokes, or other severe progressive lesions. Focal seizures often appear in people with PLEDs.

Magnetic Resonance Imaging

The most useful diagnostic tool currently available for identifying structural damage to the brain from strokes, head trauma, brain abscesses, and brain tumors is magnetic resonance imaging (MRI). This imaging technique detects disturbances in the water content of the brain, by looking at variations from region to region in the head (see Figure 9). The machine that produces these images of the brain uses magnetic fields and radio frequency waves. X-rays play no role in MRI.

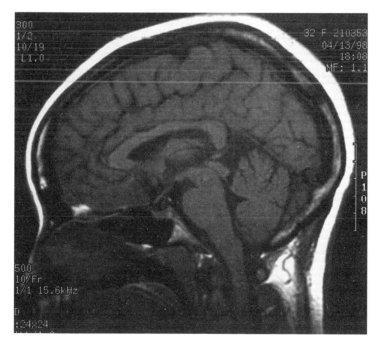

FIGURE 9. Normal MRI of the head.

Abnormal structures or changes in the normal composition of the brain can be detected on a scale of millimeters. Changes in blood flow can be observed within minutes of their development. Damage to the brain's insulating material (myelin), accumulations of fluid in the brain matter itself (edema), and shifts in the normal location of entire lobes of the brain (herniation) are easily observed with this technique. Injecting a contrast material, called gadolinium, into a vein can enhance the magnetic signature of various elements in the brain and improve the clarity of the picture provided by the MRI. This technique helps to reveal functional changes in the brain, such as local breakdowns in the blood-brain barrier, a control system found only in the brain that determines which materials are allowed to cross from the blood to the brain.

Many people with epilepsy have perfectly normal MRIs. A normal MRI does not reduce the probability of epilepsy, but it does nearly eliminate the probability that the patient's seizures are caused by a brain tumor, abscess, or other structural defect.

Conventional MRI studies cannot detect changes in the frequency of seizures or the effectiveness of antiepileptic drugs, but evolving developments in the technique may eventually change that.

Other Tools for Diagnosing Epilepsy

Computerized tomography (CT) employs imaging principles similar to those of MRI but uses x-rays to identify differences in regional densities of materials. The CT machine transmits a fine beam of x-rays through the brain and uses a computer to measure and interpret radiation absorption. The images produced by CT scanning show the brain as it would appear if it were sliced straight through at various angles. When this technique was first introduced, it greatly simplified the identification of brain tumors, abscesses, hemorrhages, and strokes.

Today, MRI has supplanted CT scanning for diagnosing these abnormalities in the so-called soft tissues, but when the fine structure of bone and other water-poor materials in the head need to be visualized, CT is still the more sensitive imaging technique.

Positron emission tomography (PET scanning) uses radio-active materials to reveal metabolic changes in the brain in very limited areas. It is primarily a research tool, and because the radioactive isotopes needed for its operation are expensive and cumbersome to produce, it will probably see much less practical application than MRI.

Strictly electrical approaches to the brain include evoked potential studies, which combine electroencephalographic techniques with computerized analysis of minute changes in brain activity. These changes are evoked in the patient by stimuli such as electrical shocks, visual patterns, or auditory clicks. The response in the brain is amplified and averaged, and a characteristic pattern can be detected.

More conventional diagnostic techniques also provide in formation on the origin of seizures. Studies of the blood and spinal fluid are usually helpful in eliminating several pos-sible causes of nervous system disease. In systemic lupus erythematosus, abnormal antibodies are apparent in the blood, and in bacterial meningitis the responsible organism is usually found in the spinal fluid. When blood vessel abnor-malities are suspected, angiography is used to visualize the vessels of the neck and head. Until a few years ago, a catheter to inject radiographic dye had to be introduced directly into the major arteries to the head, a procedure involving small but real risks. Less invasive but technologically much more com-plex is magnetic resonance angiography (MRA), a technique which uses magnetic resonance imaging to track blood flow through the brain. The principal disadvantage of MRA is that all the blood vessels, not just those of interest, in a particular region are visualized simultaneously.

Origin of Seizures

Seizure disorders may develop from obvious central nervous system injury or disease (symptomatic epilepsy) or independently of any apparent nervous system defect (idiopathic epilepsy). Particular causes of the disorder, when they can be identified, are more or less likely depending on the person's age. Some causes of epilepsy are specific for a particular age. In newborns, birth asphyxia and hereditary metabolic problems are often responsible for seizures, whereas in children, head injuries and nervous system infections are more likely to be the cause (see Chapter 6). The middle-aged adult developing seizures for the first time often has a brain tumor or a vascular problem. Seizures at any age that are initially well controlled and later recur despite antiepileptic drugs may arise from structural brain damage: tumors, abscesses, or blood clots in or over the brain; inflammatory disorders or malformations of the blood vessels to the brain; or congenital defects in the formation of the brain.

Signs and symptoms associated with the seizure disorder often help the physician determine its precise cause. Metabolic problems are usually accompanied by impaired thinking or coordination. A rapidly progressive paralysis or speech disorder associated with an obvious infection in the ear suggests a brain abscess extending from the disease in the ear. People with certain types of abnormal pigmentation in the skin or obvious vascular abnormalities over the face (portwine nevi) are at high risk of having associated nervous system tumors.

Idiopathic Seizures

Most generalized absence (petit mal) seizures and the majority of complex partial (psychomotor) seizures develop for no apparent reason. Generalized tonic-clonic (grand mal) seizures may appear after major head trauma or a central nervous system infection, but more often they too develop without any obvious cause. In many cases, examination of the brain at autopsy of someone who had epilepsy all his life will reveal no abnormalities that could account for the seizure disorder.

People whose seizures are not explained by structural damage to the brain or metabolic defects in the nervous system are assumed to have subtle problems at the level of interactions between small areas of the brain or even between individual nerve cells. Much of the brain's normal activity is inhibitory—that is, it stops miscommunication among the millions of nerve cells in the brain. Impaired function in a part of the brain that would normally dampen an electrical signal could allow unintended signals to reach another part of the brain and, once there, cause seizures.

The idea that idiopathic seizures are caused by damage to the brain before or during birth has been popular for several decades, but it is controversial and difficult to prove.

Post-traumatic Seizures

Head injuries can cause substantial brain damage and are a common cause of seizures in both children and adults. Seizures occurring at the time of an injury, called impact seizures, are an indication that the head trauma is severe. Any time that head trauma produces paralysis of an arm, loss of vision in one visual field, loss of sensation over one side of the body, skull fracture, loss of consciousness, or obvious brain damage, seizures may be a delayed effect of the injury.

When the injury to the brain is slight and no obvious tissue damage has occurred, the injury is called a concussion. People who have had concussions usually complain of headache, may have some temporary difficulty with memory, and often have lingering dizziness and sleep disorders, but epilepsy usually does not develop. With more serious injury, the brain may be bruised and swell from the pooling of tissue fluids and blood (see Figure 10). In this type of injury, called a contusion, the risk of later developing a seizure disorder is substan-

TABLE 24

Factors Increasing the Risk of Post-traumatic Epilepsy

MRI or CT evidence of cerebral contusion

Intracranial hematoma

Impact seizures

Depressed skull fracture

Tear in the dura mater lining the brain

Post-traumatic amnesia of more than 24 hours

Focal neurologic signs

tial (see Table 24). A contusion can occur even when the skull is not fractured, but trauma sufficient to produce a contusion often fractures the skull. The victim of the trauma will usually lose consciousness for more than five minutes after the impact. Memory of the episode and even of events immediately preceding the episode will be defective. Weakness in a limb, speech problems, double vision, vertigo, and changes in sensitivity to pain may occur. The extent to which these focal neurologic deficits will resolve depends on the size and location of the contusion.

Postinfectious Seizures

An infection of the brain itself is called encephalitis; an infection primarily affecting the membranes surrounding the brain and spinal cord is called meningitis. Meningitis and encephalitis frequently cause seizures when they are active, and even after the infection clears up the affected person faces substantial risk of developing a seizure disorder. Early in the course of the infection, a viral or bacterial encephalitis may produce a confusing picture of altered behavior, movement disorders, and partial or generalized seizures, but within days or weeks of these symptoms the more serious character of the disease is usually apparent. Fever, neck stiffness, and progressive impairment of consciousness routinely develop with the infection. The organism responsible for the infection is less important than the severity of the infection in determining the likelihood that epilepsy will develop after the person has recovered. Seizures that develop after nervous system infections are usually generalized.

Parasitic Disease

Parasites that invade the brain or deposit eggs in the brain account for a large proportion of seizure disorders in some

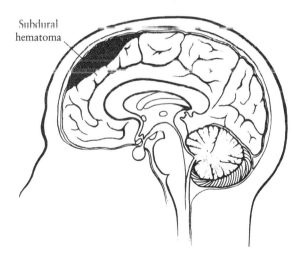

FIGURE 10. Subdural hematoma. Relatively minor trauma in elderly people can produce blood clots that overlie the brain and may produce signs of brain damage. An elderly person with confusion, weakness, and seizures may be thought to have had a stroke, but the actual problem may be a head injury that caused bleeding inside the skull.

countries. Cysticercosis from the pork tapeworm *Taenia solium* is especially common in Mexico and is often seen in the Philippines. Schistosomiasis is widespread in the less industrialized areas of East Asia, and cerebral malaria is still a frequent cause of acute seizure disorders in tropical countries. Although the parasite may not cause much damage through its own activity in the nervous system, the nervous system's reaction to the foreign agent may produce a "scar" that serves as the focus for the seizures.

Control of seizures in people with parasitic disease of the nervous system does not depend upon eradication of the parasite. Complete seizure control can be achieved even when structural damage to the brain from the parasite is obvious. The seizures that do develop may be partial or generalized.

Tumor-Related Seizures

Seizures that appear in an adult who has had no history of childhood or adolescent seizures, has suffered no trauma, is not alcoholic, has not had a stroke, and does not have an infection of the central nervous system may be caused by a tumor in the brain. These qualifications make this cause of seizures relatively infrequent simply because trauma, alcoholism, stroke, and infection are common in adults. Brain tumors are seldom the cause of seizures in childhood, because they usually occur in the brainstem and the cerebellum—areas at the base of the brain that usually do not provoke a seizure disorder when injured.

With most brain tumors, the person will have weakness in an arm or leg, sensory loss, or psychological changes as well as seizures, but even when none of these other signs is present the tumor may be highly invasive. If the tumor cannot be cured, control of the seizures with antiepileptic medications may fail as the tumor extends. Seizures that develop with tumors may be partial or generalized, but usually the type will depend on the part of the brain most damaged by the growth. For example, an occipital lobe tumor may cause visual hallucinations, whereas a frontal lobe tumor may produce twitching in an arm or a leg.

Vascular Disease

A variety of transient and permanent blood vessel disorders may produce seizures as the first sign of disease or may allow seizures to develop long after they have done considerable damage in the nervous system and elsewhere. A common vascular disease that occasionally causes epilepsy is stroke. A relatively uncommon vascular disease that frequently causes seizures is systemic lupus erythematosus. The type of person affected and the problems associated with the epilepsy vary with the vascular disorder.

Stroke

A stroke is damage to the brain caused either by inadequate blood flow or by bleeding. Inadequate blood flow reduces the oxygen supply to brain cells, causing them to die. It may occur because an artery is obstructed by cholesterol deposits in the vessel wall (atherosclerosis); or small blood clots may travel from other parts of the circulatory system and lodge in a cranial artery, obstructing blood flow. In people with diseased heart valves, these clots may form on the rough surfaces of the damaged valves and then travel to the head. Bleeding into or around the brain, which occurs when a weakened blood vessel bursts, not only deprives cells further downstream of their oxygen supply but also directly injures nearby brain tissue.

Structural brain damage late in life from stroke or even from a transient drop in the level of blood oxygen may lead to generalized or partial seizures within weeks or months. Epilepsy occasionally develops years after a stroke. If it appears after a delay of months or years, other possible causes, such as a metastatic tumor or meningitis, should be eliminated as a possibility before the stroke is declared responsible for the seizures. Even when the stroke occurs shortly before the onset of seizures, it cannot simply be assumed to be the cause of the disorder. Other problems must be looked for. If none is found, the stroke will be considered the cause of the epilepsy.

Vascular Malformation

Abnormal networks of blood vessels develop in the brains of some people while the nervous system is still forming, but the vascular malformation may not be apparent until adulthood. Although the first indication of a malformation may be a lethal hemorrhage, changes associated with these vascular abnormalities are often more subtle. Vascular malformations in the brain cause changes in the pattern of blood flow that can lead to seizures even when the malformation is small. Seizures may also be caused by vascular malformations that repeatedly bleed into the brain, causing injury, or simply grow into a large mass in the head that presses on the brain.

Vasculitis

Any inflammation of blood vessels is called vasculitis. Some types of vasculitis arise from infection, some result from allergic reactions, and some are idiopathic—that is, their cause is unknown. In young adults, systemic lupus erythematosus—which can inflame blood vessels in the head and decrease blood flow to large areas of the brain—occasionally causes generalized or complex partial seizures. In 59 percent of people with lupus, the central nervous system suffers damage, but often it is reversible. Of those with central nervous system damage, 17 to 50 percent will have seizures. Psychiatric problems are also commonly associated with this inflammatory disease, and many people with seizures caused by lupus will have depression or other changes in mood that confuse the diagnostic picture.

Metabolic Disturbances

Profoundly abnormal changes in the levels of calcium, sodium, and glucose in the blood may be responsible for generalized tonic-clonic seizures in otherwise normal people. These seizures do not represent epilepsy, since they go away entirely once the metabolic abnormality is corrected. Elevated blood urea nitrogen from kidney failure and other toxic products from liver failure can also evoke seizures. When the person has abnormal blood chemistry, there are invariably other clinical signs of the metabolic problem, but they may be obscured by the seizures. Chronic metabolic disorders from hereditary metabolic diseases are less common, but they too are occasionally responsible for epilepsy. Some, like Tay-Sachs disease, are frequently checked for in newborns.

Poisoning is a type of metabolic derangement that may cause seizures. Children are particularly likely to develop generalized seizures with nervous system damage from lead poisoning. Thallium, a poison that resembles salt, and carbon monoxide, an odorless gas emitted by faulty heating systems as well as by automobiles, may cause brain damage that induces seizures at any age. Poisoning is often difficult to detect, and so a person may suffer from generalized seizures for weeks or months before other signs suggest poison as the cause of the seizures.

Seizures Related to Alcohol and Drugs

Partial and generalized seizures often develop in alcoholics because of head injuries that occur during the period of intoxication or because of withdrawal from the alcohol. Alcohol withdrawal seizures, also known as rum fits, can occur after as little as 24 hours of alcohol abuse. They occur as isolated phenomena, as well as in 4 percent of people who go on to develop delirium tremens, the acute thought disorder that affects some chronic alcoholics during periods of withdrawal.

Seizure disorders related to alcohol abuse most commonly appear after adolescence, and they are always difficult to diagnose and treat. The diagnostic difficulty arises because people who are intoxicated are especially likely to have had head injuries, and so even a person who appears several times a year with rum fits must be evaluated for a variety of brain injuries, including cerebral contusions, subdural hematomas, and post-traumatic meningitis. The treatment difficulty arises from the behavioral and biochemical characteristics of chronic alcohol abusers. Drug compliance is erratic when these patients are not intoxicated, and it breaks down entirely when they are intoxicated. Even if the medication is given on a regular basis by a family member or friend, the rate of breakdown and excretion of antiepileptic drugs is altered by chronic drinking. Phenytoin, for example, is eliminated more quickly from the system of an alcoholic than that of a normal person or that of an alcoholic with advanced cirrhosis of the liver.

Although status epilepticus—a series of closely spaced seizures—often occurs with drug withdrawal, alcoholics are at no greater risk of developing it than are other people with seizure disorders. Seizures typically occur when the level of alcohol falls, but this does not mean that a person cannot have seizures while drunk. In fact, seizures often occur while alcoholics are still very intoxicated. Presumably, shifting levels of alcohol in the brain, together with brain damage caused by long-term alcohol abuse, provoke the seizures.

A variety of other agents that are commonly used illicitly or with medical supervision can evoke seizures in susceptible people. Antidepressants, stimulants, antipsychotic medications, and sleep preparations all occasionally allow seizures to break through in susceptible people. With some medications, such as barbiturates or benzodiazepines in sleep preparations, the seizures appear when the medication is discontinued. Tricyclic antidepressants, such as imipramine (Tofranil) and amitriptyline (Elavil), and antipsychotics such as clozapine (Clozaril) and chlorpromazine (Thorazine), presumably lower the seizure threshold directly and increase the risk of seizures as the blood level of the drug rises. Meperidine (Demerol), a commonly used prescription painkiller that is often abused by health professionals, may provoke seizures at high doses.

The effects of various illicit substances on the frequency of seizures are controversial. Despite the widespread use of marijuana, cocaine, amphetamines, and methaqualone (Quaaludes) as recreational drugs in the United States, little objective study of their contribution to the incidence or control of seizure disorders has been possible. Aside from restrictions on the use of the drugs for scientific studies, a major complicating factor has been the misrepresentation of the drugs that people actually obtain through illegal sources. One young woman, whose seizures had been well controlled for more than a year despite occasional cocaine use, developed a complex partial seizure a few days after using material given to her as a present and alleged to be high-quality cocaine. She suspected that the cocaine had been mixed with an amphetamine, because it caused mood changes similar to ones she had had in the past when taking amphetamines, but what she had actually inhaled could not be determined.

Much of what is sold as cocaine is adulterated, and these unpredictable impurities are likely to be as active as the illicit drug in the mixture. Problems of adulteration occur with all illicit drugs, and for this reason even if for no other, illegal drugs present special problems for people with epilepsy. The evidence currently available suggests that stimulants such as cocaine and amphetamines can lead to acute seizures during use.

Pseudoseizures

People who do not have epilepsy, and even some who do, occasionally pretend to have seizures. These pseudoseizures or factitious seizures are contrived to gain attention and sympathy or to avoid responsibilities. Contrived seizures would have little effect if they could be recognized for what they are, but determining whether a seizure is authentic or not is difficult, even when the observer is familiar with epilepsy. Experienced neurologists correctly identify factitious seizures in only three out of four instances.

Factitious seizures occur in both children and adults. Women have them somewhat more often than men, but they are common in both sexes. They usually begin in adolescence or young adulthood. People with pseudoseizures have a much higher than average incidence of psychiatric disease, including depressive illnesses and suicide attempts, in their families. Many also have obvious sexual problems, such as a history of sexual abuse. Although pseudoseizures are routinely called hysterical seizures or conversion reactions, terms that suggest an emotional or thought disorder, they are not necessarily caused by a psychiatric problem. They are primarily a learned response to situations and responsibilities, a technique that abruptly shifts control into the hands of the person having the attack. They can be a powerful tool with which to manipulate family, friends, and unsuspecting strangers.

Pseudoseizures have their disadvantages as well. The person who has them is unnecessarily exposed to the risks of diagnostic tests, as well as to the side effects of antiepileptic medications on the blood, liver, kidneys, and nervous system. Diane, the young wife of a busy and successful executive, had increasingly frequent generalized convulsions that resisted all antiepileptic therapy. She and her husband agreed to highly invasive studies of the brain and even to brain surgery if necessary as a last effort to control the seizures. On the transcontinental flight to the diagnostic center where further tests would be conducted and the surgery, if necessary, would be performed, she had seizures that abated only with massive doses of intravenous medication. Her husband was constantly at her side throughout the ordeal.

Extensive testing at the diagnostic center revealed no true seizures. Diane's pseudoseizures had gained her an extraordinary amount of attention from her family and physicians, but the diagnostic studies justified by the apparently life-threatening severity of her seizure disorder would have exposed her to risks that were unjustifiable in the assessment of what proved to be a psychiatric problem.

If the family realizes the attacks are contrived, the person who has developed pseudoseizures to avoid conflict may find himself embroiled even more deeply in conflict. The person's "seizures" may become more severe as the family tries to discredit the epilepsy as a real problem. If the family does not know that the seizures are contrived, considerable time and effort may be spent in a futile attempt to suppress them.

Clinical Features of Pseudoseizures

As a general rule, people who do not have epilepsy should not be exposed to the risks of antiepileptic medication, and anyone who contrives fits to make life simpler needs psychiatric help to develop less destructive techniques for dealing with friends and family. Since many people with pseudoseizures are not medically sophisticated, their seizures often display characteristics that make their authenticity questionable. Before abandoning attempts to control the seizures with medication, the physician must be very sure the episodes are contrived. Establishing this is often quite difficult even with the help of monitors of brain electrical activity. However, there are some reliable principles to follow in determining whether seizures are authentic.

Factitious seizures, like true seizures, have characteristics that appear repeatedly. In each person with pseudoseizures, the same symptoms and behavior may occur in the same sequence with each episode. The pattern that pseudoseizures assume varies somewhat with different cultures and historical periods, but the similarity is more striking than the variability.

During the nineteenth century, animal-like movements were common; currently the most common type of pseudoseizure involves limb movements with grimacing, posturing of the limbs or trunk, trembling, limb jerking, and limb flailing.

Over 80 percent have abnormal movements, and 70 percent complain of nausea, cramps, abdominal pain, bad tastes, or other symptoms related to the mouth or gastrointestinal tract—symptoms that are similar to complex partial seizures. About one-third have an apparent change in their breathing patterns, and nearly half speak, grunt, moan, sob, cough, hum, or make other types of nonverbal noises during the attack. Three out of four people with pseudoseizures make no response or bizarre responses to verbal stimuli during their fits. Dizziness, head pain, visual changes, feelings of depersonalization, hot flashes, auditory changes, and other less easily described total-body changes may occur before, during, or after the attack. Semipurposeful behavior is evident in more than half of people having a pseudoseizure, but violence is rare. The person may run, cry, make obscene gestures, chew purposelessly, choke, gag, lick or smack his lips, and hyperventilate. These abnormal behaviors usually last longer than similar phenomena occurring in true seizures.

As should be apparent from this list of symptoms, a pseudoseizure is difficult to distinguish from a complex partial seizure unless the person is attached to an electroencephalograph at the time of the episode. More helpful than what happens during the seizure is what happens after it. As in many authentic complex partial seizures, the person's abnormal movements may include or progress to tonic-clonic limb and body movements, but unlike the victim of an authentic seizure, the unsophisticated person with pseudoseizures may respond purposefully and talk within seconds of the tonic-clonic phase of a lengthy pseudoseizure. There is no postictal phase after the movements cease. The person may open his eyes and report, "I had a fit," or simply look around with surprise and ask, "What was that?"

People rarely suffer injuries during contrived fits, and only the most sophisticated patients will urinate during these episodes. Most will resist any efforts to interfere with their breathing during the ictal phase. This contrasts dramatically with the severe difficulty in breathing that some people suffer during true seizures without making any effort to clear the airway.

If all of a person's attacks are contrived, an EEG obtained during a seizure will usually indicate that it is factitious. The record will be normal except for the electrical activity generated by muscle activity as the person moves about. But obtaining such a recording to rule out true seizures may be impossible with a sophisticated person. One way to make pseudoseizures easier to detect is to use tape-recording equipment that goes everywhere with the person. Continuous monitoring of the person, especially if combined with videotaping, makes it possible to observe and analyze several episodes. By studying these recurrent episodes, the physician can usually tell whether they are authentic.

Pseudoseizures in People with Epilepsy

People who have had true seizures for several years are best able to contrive seizures, but these are precisely the people who must be assumed to be having true seizures until evidence of pseudoseizures is overwhelming. Of people with intractable seizures, 8 to 20 percent have pseudoseizures as well as true seizures. Factitious seizures occur in people with all types of epileptic disorders. A history of psychologic problems is often lacking, and family and others involved with the person are therefore obliged to assume the seizures are authentic. Any secondary gain provided by the pseudoseizures is usually fairly obvious, but the fact that the person gains something from the seizures does not prove that the seizures are contrived.

Detecting pseudoseizures in a person who also has true seizures is complicated by the fact that about 90 percent of people with epilepsy show abnormal brain waves on the EEG not just during a seizure but during the interval between true seizures. Therefore an abnormal EEG obtained during or shortly after an attack in a person with epilepsy tells the physician nothing about whether that attack was a real seizure or a pseudoseizure. Several normal records obtained shortly after attacks suggest that the person has a contrived seizure disorder, as well as a real one.

Pseudoseizures in Family Members

Contrived seizures occasionally appear in relatives of a person with epilepsy. In fact, family members who have witnessed authentic seizures may imitate them very convincingly. Children are especially likely to reenact the seizures they observe in their parents or siblings. Factitious epilepsy becomes a game for some children, or a way of getting their share of attention.

Adults rarely imitate the seizures exhibited by one of their children. Because close relatives of a person with epilepsy are at higher risk of developing seizures than the general population, any seizures in siblings or children of people with epilepsy must be considered authentic until evidence to the contrary is overwhelming.

Coping with Pseudoseizures

Contrived or factitious seizures present special problems for the family. In fact, this is one type of seizure disorder that is a much bigger problem for family members than for the affected person himself. The contrived seizure is used to gain attention or special consideration, and so it is especially difficult to suppress. Antiepileptic medication will not affect the frequency and disruptiveness of the attacks until the person is heavily sedated. Confronting the person with evidence that the seizures are not authentic will not stop the behavior but will undermine the relationship between the physician unmasking the factitious complaint and the patient.

People who have authentic seizures may develop pseudoseizures when they recognize that having a seizure exempts them from a variety of responsibilities and expectations. Reenacting the entire seizure scenario is occasionally helpful in determining what is prompting pseudoseizures. The person is asked to re-create as much as possible the activity typical of a seizure, and the rest of the family is asked to behave as it customarily does when one occurs. Without the excitement and anxiety of a real episode, the role played by each member of the family becomes more apparent, and what the person stands to gain by faking a seizure is more easily determined.

It may be possible to discourage the pseudoseizures by simple devices, such as requiring that every member of the family, not just the ones who would ordinarily care for the patient, go to the scene when a contrived seizure begins. For example, a child whose pseudoseizures in the middle of the night have always given her the exclusive attention of her father may find little incentive to have them when the entire family waits by her bed.

In any approach to pseudoseizures, a vigilance must be maintained that will not allow the person to suffer an injury even if the seizure is authentic. With this vigilance must come an evenhanded approach to the person whenever he or she appears sick. The seizure, whether real or contrived, may exempt the person from responsibilities, such as going to work or to school, but it does not entitle him or her to indulge in leisure activities. After a true seizure a person may be content to do virtually nothing for several hours, but after a contrived seizure this imposed inactivity may be intolerable. The child who cannot go to school should not be allowed to play games or watch television. It is unwise to make life with seizures entertaining when there is reason to suspect that the seizures are factitious. These seizures should be treated as unfortunate interruptions of the activities planned by the family and not as reasons for canceling plans.

Once steps have been taken to make the drama surrounding the pseudoseizure less rewarding, the person should be given a reasonable and face-saving way out. Strategies available to the patient's physician are a change in medication for a person who has real seizures as well as contrived ones, suggestions that the problem is resolving itself as a part of its natural course, and information on biofeedback techniques to modify the sensations preceding a pseudoseizure. The family plays an invaluable role in ending this type of behavior by constantly working to make it unrewarding.

Chapter Eleven

Treatment Options

Seizures are treated with a variety of techniques. Some treatment strategies involve environmental or dietary manipulation, most involve medications, and a few involve surgery. What therapy is most appropriate depends primarily on the type of seizures the person has and the history of the seizure disorder up to the time the therapy is being chosen. If only one seizure has ever occurred and if a specific stress such as protracted sleep deprivation can be identified, the physician may decide to provide no treatment other than advice on maintaining good sleep habits. At the other extreme, if the person has had seizures for years that have been uncontrolled by antiepileptic medications and is totally disabled by the seizures, surgery to remove the part of the brain thought to be the source of the seizures may be an appropriate choice for the patient and family to make.

A variety of antiepileptic drugs should be tried before surgery is considered. Most people will be free or almost free of seizures if they take the appropriate drugs. Many will continue to have frequent seizures, but the severity of their disorder will not be great enough to justify surgery. The decision to take out part of someone's brain should be reached only after other reasonable options have been exhausted. The negative effects of this surgery are irreversible, and there are no guarantees that the person will accrue long-term or even short-term benefits. As surgical techniques and medication options keep changing, physicians, their patients, and family members must constantly revise their thinking about who is an appropriate candidate for brain surgery.

Being free of seizures means having the opportunity to lead a relatively normal life. Incomplete control that develops after a long seizure-free period can often be traced to changes in the patient's lifestyle, general health, or level of compliance. If a person has had good seizure control with a single antiepileptic drug or a combination of drugs, it is likely the person will be able to return to good seizure control with relatively minor changes in medications or lifestyle.

Unfortunately, some people have persistently poor seizure control despite appropriate modifications in their personal habits, drug dose, and willingness to cooperate. For a few, recurrent or refractory seizures are a sign of new or extended disease of the central nervous system. For others, the intractable seizures have no explanation or treatable cause and provide a constant source of frustration and despair.

No case of intractable seizures should be considered hopeless just because currently available treatments are ineffective. New drugs are being tested and introduced every year. This search for better drugs continues even though the antiepileptic medications now available can eliminate or decrease the frequency of most types of seizures. Researchers continue to seek drugs that can be taken fewer times a day and that can suppress seizures without causing side effects such as allergic reactions, gastrointestinal distress, lethargy, impotence, or confusion. Side effects limit the usefulness of all of the antiepileptic drugs now available. Some people are unable to take the medication that is most effective for their type of seizure disorder because they cannot tolerate the adverse reactions. Fortunately, with most of the drugs used, the side effects are relatively minor, considering the independence and security they provide.

For people with seizures that do not respond to medications, alternative treatments may include surgery and dietary approaches. But regardless of what type of treatment the person with epilepsy receives, getting in touch with other people who have similar problems is usually helpful. Meetings of similarly affected families can reduce frustrations, especially when seizure control is poor, by providing new perspectives and strategies. Patients are often more frank with other patients than with their physician. They do not want to alienate their doctor by confessing medication lapses or experimentation with alternative therapies, because they may need the doctor's help in the future. But when they talk to other people with epilepsy and their families, they have little reason to gloss over these sensitive topics.

Antiepileptic Drugs

Most people with epilepsy have fewer or less severe seizures when they take antiepileptic medication (see Table 25). How well a person will respond to drugs is affected by the type of central nervous system damage that is causing the epilepsy, the person's ability to absorb and metabolize the drugs, any nonneurologic problems that may be associated with the epilepsy, and the patient's compliance with medication instructions. Despite these and many other variables, the likelihood that a particular person will do well on medication is fairly predictable.

The people who respond best to drugs are those with idiopathic epilepsy—that is, those with no apparent explanation for their seizure disorders, such as an old head injury or meningitis (see Table 26). A second predictor is the frequency of

TABLE 25
Generic and Brand Names of Antiepileptic Drugs

Drug	Brand
Carbamazepine	Tegretol
Clonazepam	Klonopin
Ethosuximide	Zarontin
Felbamate	Felbatol
Gabapentin	Neurontin
Lamotrigine	Lamictal
Lorazepam	Ativan
Phenobarbital	(numerous)
Phenytoin	Dilantin
Valproate (divalproex)	Depakote
Valproic acid	Depakene

seizures before starting medication: the less frequent the seizure episodes, the better the level of control that can be achieved. The patient's age also affects the likelihood of complete seizure control with medication: seizures that appear before age 10 are generally more easily controlled than those that appear later. But if seizures begin in the child's first year of life, the outlook is poor. An important exception to this rule is simple febrile seizures, which are common in infants and do not indicate long-term epilepsy. The poor outcome when other types of seizures appear before one year of age is probably due to the high probability of congenital brain damage in this group of infants. An especially worrisome sign is the association of a profoundly abnormal electroencephalogram (hypsarrhythmia) with associated body and limb jerks

TABLE 26

Outlook for Complete Seizure Control

Good	Poor
Strictly generalized seizures	Complex partial seizures with tonic-clonic activity as well
Idiopathic seizures	Seizures caused by contusion, tumor, stroke, meningitis, etc.
No cognitive impairment	Cognitive abilities impaired
No personality disorder	Obvious personality disorder
Normal EEG or minor background abnormalities	Anterior temporal or frontal lobe abnormalities on EEG
Onset between 1 and 5 years of age	Onset before 1 year of age

(infantile spasms). Even with early treatment, the outlook for seizure control and normal cognitive development in these children is poor.

Good seizure control is most easily achieved in people who start taking antiepileptic drugs within a year of their first seizure. Epilepsy is more likely to be fully controlled if it is treated early and aggressively than if it is allowed to recur in the hope that the person will grow out of it without treatment. Of people who remain free of seizures during their first year of treatment, 87 percent will have no seizures for at least three years if they continue the treatment.

Seizure control is more elusive if the person has more than one type of seizure, a grossly abnormal neurologic examination, signs of mental retardation or low IQ, or a severe personality disorder. Electrical studies of the brain can sometimes help detect people who are likely to respond poorly to antiepileptic medication, but the patient's history is usually more predictive of seizure control on medication than any specific pattern on the EEG. Epilepsy that develops after a massive head injury, for example, is not likely to remit completely on any antiepileptic regimen. People whose seizures are caused by strokes or central nervous system infections, on the other hand, usually achieve good control with a single antiepileptic drug.

Probably the most important factor in determining the level of seizure control that will be possible is the type of seizure disorder the person has. With appropriate antiepileptic therapy, complete elimination of seizures is possible in about 60 percent of people with partial seizures. This relatively high level of control occurs in people with both simple (focal motor, focal sensory) and some types of complex partial seizures.

With generalized tonic-clonic (grand mal) seizures, complete control is feasible in more than 70 percent of people treated with the best drugs currently available. This is about the same level of control that can be achieved in generalized absence (petit mal) seizures. Taking all seizure types together, only about 9 percent of people on standard antiepileptic treatment show no response to the drugs, and at least 58 percent have complete seizure control.

The EEG may remain distinctly abnormal even while a person is seizure-free. Improvement in seizure control usually precedes improvement in the pattern of a person's brain waves. Even when an abnormal EEG persists for years after the seizures begin, this pattern is not a good predictor of future seizures. On the other hand, abnormal brain wave patterns shortly after the first seizure often do predict more seizures. Antiepileptic drugs may return the person to a normal level of functioning even though the brain has obvious electrical abnormalities.

Initiating Drug Treatment

For most people, antiepileptic treatment should be attempted initially with a single drug. This is called monotherapy. About

60 percent of people with recurrent seizures achieve good control on one antiepileptic drug. Nearly half of these are controlled on phenytoin (Dilantin) alone; about a third use carbamazepine (Tegretol) alone; and about one-eighth are on valproate (Depakote; see descriptions of these drugs below). Control with valproate alone would probably be similar to that seen with phenytoin if valproate were used as commonly as phenytoin.

For each seizure type and for each epilepsy syndrome there is one or a few drugs of choice that should be used in monotherapy, unless something in the history suggests that the patient will not tolerate it. If the first-line drug fails to achieve seizure control, alternative drugs known to suppress the seizure type that persists should be tried in combination with the first-line drug. If complete seizure control develops with the addition of a second-line drug, it may be practical to gradually withdraw the ineffective first-line drug. Ideally, a person should achieve complete seizure control on the fewest drugs possible.

That ideal cannot always be met, however. About 30 percent of people with epilepsy who take medication require a combination of drugs to control their seizures. Some people will exhibit poor or incomplete seizure control with both first-line and alternative drugs. In those cases, drugs that have been tested and have demonstrated effectiveness in combination with first- or second-line drugs may be added on to improve overall seizure control. Sometimes three drugs must be used in people with refractory epilepsy, although the incremental benefit tends to diminish with each drug added. Many of the drugs currently approved for use as add-on medications, such as felbamate (Felbatol), lamotrigine (Lamictal), topiramate (Topamax), and gabapentin (Neurontin), have also been used alone and have shown a high level of efficacy; in the future they may be used in monotherapy as well.

How a given drug regimen is started in a given person depends on the drug and on the person. Some, such as phenytoin, may be started with a loading dose of 500 mg on the first day of treatment. Others, such as carbamazepine, topiramate, tiagabine (Gabatril), lamotrigine, and perhaps gabapentin, must be introduced at a fraction of the dose the person will eventually be able to tolerate and must be increased to the maximum tolerated or maximally effective dose over the course of weeks. If the drug is being added to another antiepileptic medication, how the two drugs will interact must be considered in setting the initial dose and dose escalation. For example, lamotrigine added to valproate must be introduced at about one-quarter the dose normally tolerated by people not already on valproate.

Any treatment adopted must consider the specific circumstances of the patient. Just as diagnostic methods must take into consideration the patient's age, so too must treatment. The newborn with seizures may have vitamin B6 (pyridoxine) deficiency and require emergency vitamin therapy. The adult with unexplained seizures may require detoxification from cocaine or amphetamines. If the patient is a child, adjustments in the recommended dose must be made to take into consideration the changing patterns of drug absorption and metabolism at different points in development. Interactions with other drugs or even specific features of the diet must be considered in people of all ages. The effects of antiepileptic drugs on oral contraceptives and the impact of medications on pregnancy, childbirth, and the health of the fetus are major concerns for women of childbearing age (see Chapter 5).

Follow-Up by the Physician

During a patient's first year of taking an antiepileptic drug, several follow-up visits to the physician are essential. Within a few weeks of starting medication, blood tests will show if the person is tolerating the drug and if enough is getting into the bloodstream. If seizure control is poor or side effects are a problem, the dose or type of drug may need to be changed.

The more closely people are followed by physicians after drug treatment is started, the better their seizure control usually is. People who are willing to see a doctor are often also willing to comply with the doctor's instructions. When seizure control is poor, the person is more likely to be skeptical of the treatment and to experiment with unorthodox therapies. Despite the reluctance of those most in need of supervision—those whose seizure control is poor—to submit to it, a substantial improvement in control can often be achieved if the physician makes a concerted effort to monitor the person directly or with the cooperation of the family.

During follow-up visits, the physician has an opportunity to see if any new information about the cause of the seizure disorder has surfaced. The physician can also reinforce instructions on taking the medication and answer the patient's or family's questions under circumstances that are less stressful than those of the first visit. When seizure control is complete, follow-up examinations by a doctor familiar with the problem may be necessary only once a year. If any dramatic changes in health or lifestyle occur, however, the physician should be consulted to see if any adjustments in antiepileptic medication are needed.

Recurrent seizures in people whose seizures previously have been well-controlled on an antiepileptic drug often result from failure to take the drug as prescribed. A physician should never assume that poor compliance is the only problem when seizures recur, but the probability is high that it is a factor. A check of antiepileptic drug levels in the blood and a routine reevaluation of the patient's overall health status are appropriate when seizure control has deteriorated.

What constitutes responsible monitoring by the physician in the weeks and months following the first visit is determined by the patient's age, general condition and competence, level of seizure control, treatment regimen, and childbearing interests. When antiepileptic drugs are first introduced, supervision by the physician is necessarily more rigorous. Antiepileptic drug levels will usually be measured to help establish that the person is taking the prescribed medication properly and to identify drug interactions. How often blood counts, liver function tests, and other blood parameters are measured will depend on the individual drugs and drug combinations being used. Carbamazepine may depress the white blood cell count but rarely causes severe suppression of the bone marrow where blood forms. Felbamate, on the other hand, can cause a fatal anemia as a consequence of bone marrow suppression and is sometimes associated with liver failure. These risks dictate the routine testing that will be ordered.

In most cases, physicians will order blood counts, liver function tests, and measurements of antiepileptic drug levels every two to four weeks over the first two months and every one to two months for the subsequent six months. This follow-up strategy should establish whether the person can tolerate the drug and is handling it as expected. After that, testing may be reduced to once every three months or less often as uneventful years pass. People whose seizure disorder is well controlled and whose blood tests are unremarkable should be assessed once or twice a year. Women who are pregnant or considering pregnancy require monitoring on a monthly or, late in the pregnancy, weekly basis (see Chapter 5).

Medication Options

Phenobarbital was introduced in 1912 and provided dramatic relief from seizures for many people. Its inability to suppress all seizure types and its side effects, primarily sedation in adults and hyperactivity in children, prompted the development of other antiepileptics.

Phenytoin (Dilantin) entered clinical neurology in 1938 and immediately became the gold standard by which all other antiepileptics were measured. Most of the antiepileptics subsequently developed had chemical ties to phenobarbital and phenytoin. Primidone (Mysoline) was so closely related to phenobarbital that when it was first introduced there was controversy over whether its only active metabolite was phenobarbital. Ethosuximide (Zarontin) and methsuximide (Celontin) had no advantages over phenytoin in most seizure disorders, but they proved more effective than other drugs in suppressing generalized absence (petit mal) seizures. Valproate (Depakote) is one of the few older antiepileptic drugs with no structural similarity to phenobarbital or phenytoin. It has proved valuable in treating generalized as well as partial seizure disorders, but it has disadvantages, such as increased appetite, hair loss, and weight gain.

In order to be effective, antiepileptic drugs, like other drugs, must reach a "therapeutic level"—a concentration of the drug in the blood serum that causes few or no side effects and gives maximum benefit to most patients who respond to the drug. This is usually measured in micrograms (μg) per milliliter (mL) of blood serum and is different for every drug. How much medication will produce a therapeutic level, in turn, varies from individual to individual. If a person is responding poorly to a conventional dose of antiepileptic medication, the physician should check the level of the drug in the blood to make sure that it is in the therapeutic range. One must keep in mind, however, that different patients may respond quite differently even to the same blood level of a given drug.

All of the currently used antiepileptic drugs have side effects. Most of the risks are the same for all people taking a given medication, but there are noteworthy exceptions. Women trying to become pregnant while taking antiepileptics must face the risk of birth defects (see Chapter 5). Some men may find that certain drugs, such as phenobarbital, make them impotent. People with chronic liver disease or alcoholism may not be able to tolerate drugs metabolized in the liver. The risk of unwanted side effects is minimized by using the antiepileptics that are most effective against the patient's seizure type (see Table 27).

Over the past decade several new drugs have been intro-

TABLE 27

Antiepileptic Drugs of Choice

Seizure type	First line	Alternatives	Add-ons
Generalized tonic-clonic	Valproate	Phenytoin Carbamazepine Lamotrigine	Gabapentin Phenobarbital Lamotrigine
Complex partial	Carbamazepine Phenytoin	Valproate Felbamate	Topiramate Tiagabine Gabapentin Lamotrigine
Generalized absence	Ethosuximide	Valproate	Lamotrigine Clonazepam
Atypical absence	Valproate	Phenytoin	Clonazepam
Simple partial	Carbamazepine Phenytoin		Topiramate Tiagabine Gabapentin Lamotrigine
Complex febrile	Valproate	Phenobarbital Primidone	Phenytoin
Generalized myoclonic	Valproate		Clonazepam
Infantile spasms	Adrenocortico-tropic hormone	Valproate Nitrazepam	Clonazepam Primidone

duced whose effectiveness in suppressing seizures seems established but whose long-term adverse health effects remain to be determined. Vigabatrin has demonstrated some value in cases of infantile spasms, a difficult-to-treat condition; in Europe it is also prescribed for partial seizures, but it is believed to cause damage to the retina of the eye and other nerve tissue and so is generally considered unacceptable as a first-line or adjunctive therapy in the United States. Questions of safety have also been raised for lamotrigine (Lamictal), topiramate (Topamax), tiagabine (Gabatril), and particularly felbamate (Felbatol). Felbamate can suppress bone marrow production and very rarely cause liver failure. With topiramate, many people complain of problems with memory or other disturbances of thinking.

Phenytoin (Dilantin)

For several decades, phenytoin (Dilantin, Epanutin) has proven its relative safety and effectiveness in the treatment of a wide range of seizure types, including some partial seizure disorders and seizures developing after brain surgery and head trauma. Its popularity is largely due to the fact that it can be administered intravenously when necessary and it is not sedating. For generalized tonic-clonic (grand mal) seizures, phenytoin is commonly the first drug prescribed, even though valproate is a more appropriate first choice.

Phenytoin is usually supplied as a capsule (100 milligrams), tablet (50 mg), or syrup and is given in one or more doses daily. The average adult dose required to maintain a therapeutic level of the drug in the blood is 300–400 mg daily, usually taken in three or four capsules. A therapeutic level of 10–20 μg/mL of blood serum c\an be reached in four to ten hours. Children can usually tolerate 4–7 mg of phenytoin per kilogram (kg) of body weight per day, and good levels in children can usually be maintained with one dose per day.

An adult being introduced to the drug for the first time, or after serum drug levels have dropped to negligible levels, may be given up to 1,000 mg of phenytoin by mouth per day until a therapeutic level is reached. As long as the concentration of the drug in the blood remains less than 10 μg/mL, the physician will assume that an effective level of the drug has not yet been achieved. If the blood concentration of phenytoin shoots past 20 μg/mL, the physician will be concerned about side effects.

Reaching a therapeutic level of any drug by mouth is usually a slow process that takes days rather than hours. In an emergency, phenytoin can also be administered intravenously to both children and adults, and therapeutic levels of the drug can be reached within minutes. But because of the small risk of irritating the heart, IV phenytoin is not advisable except when a person is actively seizing and when reaching a therapeutic level quickly may be life-saving.

Recently fosphenytoin (Cerebyx) has been approved as an alternative to intravenous phenytoin. It is effective when given through intramuscular injection (which phenytoin is not), and it is less irritating to the veins when administered intravenously. It is also safer to give intravenously than is phenytoin. Fosphenytoin is converted to phenytoin after it is absorbed or injected intravenously.

Side Effects

Although phenytoin occasionally produces blood disorders and allergic reactions, the more common serious reactions are neurologic and psychologic. A staggering gait, slurred speech, blurred vision, and mild sedation are the most frequent complaints, especially at high levels, though many people experience none of these side effects. Some people complain that the drug upsets their stomach or alters bowel patterns, but these problems are usually mild and transient. Decades of phenytoin use often cause persistent but mild gait problems and sensory loss. These result from injury to peripheral nerves and nervous system centers for balance control.

The most disturbing side effect of phenytoin is its cosmetic effect. Women in particular complain that their facial features become coarser and the hair on their face and limbs gets darker. Aggravation of acne is also a common complaint. Both men and women are frequently plagued by an overgrowth of the gums (gingival hyperplasia), which is unsightly and can lead to tooth loss.

Psychologic problems rarely occur as adverse reactions to

phenytoin, but the range of psychologic reactions that do occur is broad. Many people complain of cognitive slowing and poor concentration, and a very few people have hallucinations. Confusion and disorientation are especially common in people who had minor problems in memory or thinking before taking the medication. The person on phenytoin may report difficulty with memory or calculations, and family or friends may find the person irascible.

These complications may actually be caused by other drugs taken simultaneously that interfere with the breakdown of phenytoin, including diazepam (Valium), chlorpromazine (Thorazine), prochlorperazine (Compazine), methylphenidate (Ritalin), cimetidine (Tagamet), and chlordiazepoxide (Librium).

If a person develops a rash shortly after starting phenytoin, an allergy to the drug is assumed to be responsible, and the drug will be stopped. Many people develop new complaints, such as blurred vision or tremors, that may come from too high a level of phenytoin in the blood or from a problem unrelated to phenytoin. The simplest way to check for phenytoin toxicity is to obtain a blood serum level.

The level of phenytoin in the blood should reach a plateau after the person has been on oral doses of the drug for about five days. With serum levels higher than 20 μg/mL, toxic signs may appear and seizures may even get worse. Toxic effects other than acute allergic or gastrointestinal reactions should not arise for several hours after taking the drug by mouth, because absorption is slow and peak blood levels are not reached until four to ten hours after an oral dose. Because phenytoin is metabolized primarily in the liver, people with impaired liver function may reach toxic concentrations of the drug more readily than other people. Impaired kidney function may also increase the risk of toxicity.

Attempts to commit suicide by taking an overdose of phenytoin are usually unsuccessful, because irritation of the stomach will trigger vomiting of a massive oral dose. Most people find it difficult to take more than 500 mg (five capsules) at one time. In fact, many people with no interest in committing suicide are limited in the number of tablets or capsules they can take at once, because of stomach irritation and the nausea and vomiting that it may evoke. If more than ten or fifteen capsules are swallowed and retained, the principal danger of the drug is in its cardiac action, though fatal arrhythmias rarely occur even after such massive oral doses. A rapid intravenous infusion of phenytoin carries a risk of cardiac arrest, but most people do not have the means to inject the medication directly into the bloodstream, and phenytoin injected into muscle is very poorly absorbed.

Any woman of childbearing age taking this drug faces the risk of birth defects should she become pregnant, but the increase in risk over that associated with merely having epilepsy is relatively slight. The types of birth defects include cleft palate, skeletal anomalies, and holes (septal defects) between chambers of the heart. Some of the birth defects may be a consequence of reductions in the level of the vitamin folate induced by phenytoin. Phenytoin also interferes with the level of vitamin K in the body. Women who are taking phenytoin should supplement their diet with vitamin K during the last months of pregnancy and with folate throughout pregnancy. If they are planning to become pregnant they should start taking folate supplements at least a few months prior to conception.

Abnormal liver function, disturbed immune response, depressed vitamin B12 or folic acid levels, interference with vitamin D metabolism, and altered (though inconsequential) thyroid function are all possible consequences of phenytoin use. These parameters should be monitored and managed if disturbed. If phenytoin must be stopped, it may be discontinued abruptly, but people at risk for seizures should be treated with an alternative antiepileptic medication to prevent recurrent seizures or status epilepticus. Drug interactions are likely when replacement therapy is started before phenytoin has been cleared by the body, and levels of the new drug may fluctuate until phenytoin is out of the bloodstream.

Valproate (Depakote, Depakene)

Valproate, valproic acid (Depakene), and divalproex sodium (Depakote) are different forms of dipropylacetic acid and its salts, all of which deliver valproate as an antiepileptic agent to the blood. Valproate has proven extremely effective against several different types of generalized as well as partial seizures and has been well-tolerated by both children and adults. It is the drug of choice for atypical absence seizures and atonic seizures, and it is useful against myoclonic photosensitive seizures, other myoclonic seizures, complex febrile seizures, and absence seizures associated with generalized tonic-clonic seizures. It has also been useful in controlling complex partial seizures that have been difficult to control with more conventional drugs, such as carbamazepine (Tegretol).

Divalproex sodium can be administered as a 250 or 500 mg tablet, a 125 mg sprinkle capsule, or a 500 mg slow-release tablet. Valproic acid is available as a syrup (50 mg/5 mL) and as a 250 mg tablet. Adults usually require 1–3 grams per day to maintain therapeutic levels. Children typically require 15–18 mg/kg of body weight per day.

An intravenous preparation of valproic acid—Depakon—is available for in-hospital use. This allows people to receive the drug when they cannot take any drug by mouth or when therapeutic levels must be reached in minutes or hours instead of days or weeks.

Most people's seizures can be controlled with 3 or 4 (or occasionally as few as 2) evenly spaced doses of valproate daily. Whenever valproate is used in combination with other drugs, blood tests should be done to establish that the amount of drug in the blood is not drifting out of the therapeutic range. For most people the therapeutic level of valproate is 50–100 µg/mL, but some people require 125 µg/mL or more and can tolerate this level without substantial side effects. Combining valproate with clonazepam (Klonopin) heightens the risk of absence status epilepticus.

Side Effects

Valproate may produce gastrointestinal upset even when it is given as a coated tablet. This can be minimized by taking it with meals. Less common side effects include drowsiness, hair loss, weight gain, and elevated liver enzymes. Much more rarely, people may have changes in blood components, such as the platelets involved in clotting. Tremors, bedwetting, insomnia, headache, and loss of appetite develop in some people. These side effects are generally reversible when the drug is stopped.

Children under two years of age have adverse liver reactions more commonly than any other group of people, but these problems are still quite rare. The children most at risk are those with congenital malformations. Unfortunately, liver damage, if it occurs, may be lethal for the infant treated with valproate. These rare liver reactions are not dose-related but are most likely to occur when valproate is used in combination with other antiepileptic drugs. Inflammation of the pancreas can occasionally develop at any age.

Women of childbearing age who take valproate are at increased risk of having children with defects in nervous system formation (such as spina bifida). The fetus is most at risk if the drug is taken during the first trimester of pregnancy. Alpha-fetoprotein screening in the first trimester can usually detect this defect. Taking supplements of folate before conception may reduce this risk.

Carbamazepine (Tegretol)

Carbamazepine is highly effective against a variety of partial seizures and generalized tonic-clonic (though not other generalized) seizures. It is the drug of choice for complex partial seizures and is useful for managing simple partial and secondarily generalized tonic-clonic seizures. Unlike other antiepileptic drugs that are effective against these seizure types, carbamazepine does not usually impair thinking and does not produce substantial sedation at therapeutic doses.

Carbamazepine comes as a 200 mg tablet or as a 100 mg chewable tablet. It is also available in an extended release form (Tegretol-XR in 100, 200, and 400 mg tablets; Carbatrol in 200 and 300 mg tablets). A liquid form (100 mg/ 5 mL of fluid) is available for children and other people unable to swallow tablets, but no intravenous preparation is available. Most adults must start with 100 mg doses to avoid stomach or intestinal discomfort. An initial dose of 100 mg two to three times daily can be advanced over the course of two to four weeks to 600–1,600 mg daily; in children, a typical dose is 20–30 mg/kg of body weight daily. The therapeutic range is 4–12 μg/mL.

Side Effects

Depression of the white blood cell count occurs frequently in people taking carbamazepine, but it is rarely of any consequence and is readily reversible by discontinuing the drug. If the white blood cell count stays above 4,000 per cubic millimeter (cmm) and the person does not have disturbed immune function, there is no reason to stop the medication. Much less commonly, a depressed platelet count may develop and must be monitored closely. Most physicians stop the drug if platelets drop below 75,000/cmm. Below 20,000/cmm, bleeding may occur.

Numerous gastrointestinal complaints develop with the drug, but they are usually transient. Children may have insomnia, agitation, irritability, and mood swings if drug levels drift above the therapeutic range. Abruptly stopping carbamazepine may precipitate rebound seizures in some people. Women of childbearing age are at slightly increased risk of birth defects in their offspring if they are on carbamazepine during their pregnancies. Neural tube defects (spina bifida) occur in 0.5–1 percent of cases.

Ethosuximide (Zarontin)

Ethosuximide is most useful against generalized absence (petit mal) attacks of childhood. It comes in 250 mg capsules or 50 mg/mL syrup and is rapidly absorbed within two to four hours. Most children can be started at 15 mg/kg of body weight per day in two or three divided doses and can be advanced at weekly intervals to 40 mg/kg/day to achieve therapeutic blood serum levels (40–100 μg/mL). Adults taking 750–2,000 mg daily will usually achieve this therapeutic level.

Side Effects
Gastrointestinal distress is not unusual when the drug is started. Some children have agitation, euphoria, apathy, night terrors, and paranoid delusions, all of which are unrelated to dose. Some people will develop rashes or low platelet counts.

Primidone (Mysoline)

Primidone is useful against complex partial (psychomotor) seizures and may be helpful for people with poorly controlled generalized tonic-clonic or myoclonic seizures. It is available as 50 or 250 mg tablets and as a 50 mg/mL syrup. Adults may take doses of 300–1,500 mg to reach a therapeutic blood serum level (6–12 μg/mL). Children usually require 10–25 mg/kg of body weight per day.

One metabolite of primidone is phenobarbital: consequently a person on a therapeutic dose of primidone may develop a toxic level of phenobarbital in the blood. For this reason, blood levels should be regularly measured. Side effects of primidone include sedation, confusion, gait unsteadiness, and clumsiness. More serious but much rarer are acute confusional states, persecutory delusions, and impotence.

Phenobarbital

From its introduction, the shortcomings of phenobarbital have been apparent. The most obvious problem with this drug is a narrow therapeutic window: the difference between the anticpileptic dose and the sedative dose is small or nonexistent. Nevertheless, the drug is still widely used, largely because many practitioners are familiar with it and feel more comfortable using it than they do using more recently introduced medications. It is also inexpensive and can be taken once a day, and it is effective for a broad range of seizure types. It is useful in contexts, such as status epilepticus, where sedation is not a concern. Adults will usually achieve therapeutic levels (15–35 μg/mL) with an oral dose of 90–200 mg/day. Similar levels are reached in children given doses of 3–5 mg/kg of body weight per day. The drug is available in 15, 30, 60, and 100 mg tablets, and in a 4 mg/mL syrup.

Many physicians mistakenly consider phenobarbital a safe drug, but its adverse side effects are numerous and serious. In addition to causing drowsiness, irritability, and mood swings, children given the drug may develop hyperactivity and aggressiveness. Children and infants on the drug for months or years may exhibit developmental delays and learning problems. Some men on the drug develop impotence. Signs of drug toxicity include slurred speech, staggering gait, and nystagmus—involuntary jerking movements of the eyes. People with the metabolic disease porphyria and people with severe depression should not be given the drug. A pregnant woman should not take the drug during the first trimester unless she was on this medication before she became pregnant. How late in pregnancy phenobarbital exerts an effect on the fetus is unknown (see Chapter 6).

Abrupt phenobarbital withdrawal may evoke rebound seizures, even in people who have never had seizures. Because it depresses respiration, an accidental or intentional overdose may be lethal. Suicide is a practical possibility among people who have access to phenobarbital. And finally, the many adverse side effects can lead patients to poor compliance.

Adrenocorticotropic Hormone (ACTH)

Although ACTH is not generally regarded as an antiepileptic medication, this hormone is highly effective in suppressing infantile spasms. It is usually administered intravenously or intramuscularly for two to three weeks. If the infant responds with fewer seizures, the hormone may be increased to achieve better control. Treatment with ACTH is rarely continued for more than two months.

Side Effects
Even when given for the short courses typically used in managing this infantile spasm, ACTH may cause sleep disturbances, increased susceptibility to infections, high blood sugar, high blood pressure, gastrointestinal ulcers, fluid retention, and rounding of the face, among other side effects.

Lamotrigine (Lamictal)

For people who cannot achieve control of complex partial seizures with one drug, lamotrigine may be effective when given as an addition to another antiepileptic medication. An obvious disadvantage of the drug is that it must be started at very low doses (12.5–50 mg daily) for two weeks before it can be increased to a maximum of 250–500 mg daily, given as two doses per day. The maximum pace at which the dose can be advanced is about 100 mg daily each week. People who are also on valproate (divalproex sodium) should be started on lamotrigine at 25 mg every other day and advanced to a maximum dose of 150 mg daily to avoid overdose. If lamotrigine must be discontinued, it is best to taper the dose over a minimum of two weeks.

Side Effects
The most common adverse effects of lamotrigine are dizziness, double vision, blurred vision, clumsiness, staggering, rash, nausea, and drowsiness.

Gabapentin (Neurontin)

Gabapentin (Neurontin) is used in people whose partial seizures persist despite treatment with other antiepileptic drugs. It is still recommended for use in conjunction with other antiepileptic drugs, but some physicians are using it alone. It comes in 100, 300, or 400 mg capsules and reaches peak plasma concentrations within two to three hours. What is the therapeutic level in an adult is not agreed upon, but good seizure control can usually be achieved with a daily dose of 900–1,800 mg. The drug should be started at 300 mg (three 100 mg capsules or one 300 mg capsule) nightly and increased to twice daily on the second day of dosing and three times daily on the third day. The dose may be escalated to as much as 800 mg three times a day over the course of a few days. The maximum recommended dose is 600 mg three times a day, but some people require and tolerate substantially higher doses. People with kidney disease should be managed with lower doses. Antacids interfere with its absorption.

Gabapentin is not metabolized in the liver and does not appear to alter the plasma level of other antiepileptics taken concurrently, such as carbamazepine, phenobarbital, phenytoin, and valproate.

Side Effects
When gabapentin is used along with other antiepileptic drugs, side effects include lethargy, dizziness, staggering gait, and disturbed eye movements (nystagmus). Whether or not the drug is safe during pregnancy or breastfeeding is unknown. It is not yet approved for use in children. Gradual reduction of the dose over the course of a week is safer than abrupt discon-

tinuation of the drug. Seizures may develop or become more frequent with abrupt withdrawal.

Felbamate (Felbatol)

Felbamate (Felbatol) has been approved for use in partial seizures, and it is also effective against a variety of seizure types associated with the childhood disturbance Lennox-Gastaut syndrome, at least when used in combination with other antiepileptic medications. The seizure types targeted by felbamate include absence, atonic, and generalized tonic-clonic seizures.

Felbamate is available in 400 and 600 mg tablets, as well as in a 120 mg/mL syrup. In adults, felbamate should be started at 300 mg orally four times a day and increased every three days by 600 mg, up to a maximum daily dose of 3,600 mg. Felbamate is well absorbed when taken by mouth, even if it is taken with food or antacids. It reaches peak levels within a few hours and is excreted in the urine after being partly metabolized in the liver to inactive metabolites. There is no consensus on what is the therapeutic range. Children can usually tolerate 30–60 mg/kg daily.

Other antiepileptic medications will usually need to be reduced as the felbamate dose increases. Without a 20 to 30 percent reduction in these other drugs, side effects will develop.

Side Effects
The most common side effects with felbamate include headache, insomnia, loss of appetite, fatigue, nausea, vomiting, weight loss, constipation, diarrhea, and gastrointestinal discomfort. Effects of the drug on pregnancy and breastfeeding are unknown.

A relatively high incidence of aplastic anemia, which is a potentially lethal disturbance of blood formation, and a high rate of liver failure have deterred physicians from prescribing this drug. The apparent incidence of aplastic anemia in people taking felbamate for several months is 1 in 3,500–5,000. About 1 in 24,000–32,000 develop fatal liver disease.

Clonazepam (Klonopin)

Clonazepam is useful primarily against myoclonic seizures, atypical absence, and atonic seizures. Therapeutic blood serum levels (.013–.072 μg/mL) can usually be maintained in adults with only 1.5–2 mg taken daily in two or three divided doses. Children can usually tolerate no more than 0.01–0.02 mg/kg of body weight per day initially, although drug tolerance after exposure for days or weeks may reach 0.2 mg/kg/day. It is available as 0.5, 1, and 2 mg tablets but not in syrup form.

Although clonazepam is used in children for Lennox-Gastaut syndrome, atypical absence, myoclonic, atonic, and absence seizures, it often causes hyperactivity, emotional instability, aggressiveness, and irritability in children. Adults often complain of drowsiness and clumsiness. For both children and adults, the likelihood of sedation limits the dose that physicians typically prescribe. Most side effects from clonazepam are dose-related and completely resolve with withdrawal of the drug, but withdrawal seizures are a possibility.

Lorazepam (Ativan)

Lorazepam is used to help manage complex partial seizures when given orally and to help manage status epilepticus when given intravenously. It is available in 1 mg tablets and may produce a therapeutic blood serum level (0.03–0.07 μg/mL) with 1–5 mg daily in two to five divided doses. Sedation is likely to limit the dose that the person can take.

Surgery

Surgical removal of a piece of brain tissue where abnormal electrical activity begins can be effective in controlling epi-

TABLE 28

Criteria for Good Surgical Candidates

IQ over 75
Highly motivated
No diffuse brain damage
MRI abnormal in one spot
Clearly defined seizure focus that can be removed without causing major neurologic deficits
Seizures uncontrolled by maximum tolerated dose of several drugs

lepsy that cannot be controlled with medication (see Table 28). But because any surgery on the brain may produce a new injury that can lead to seizures or other neurological deficits, removal of brain tissue to control seizures is usually performed as a last resort, after drug treatment has failed. The procedure is feasible only when a distinct piece of brain tissue that is causing the seizures can be identified and when removal of the tissue will not cause unacceptable weakness, memory loss, speech difficulty, or other problems. This means, for example, that if abnormal electrical activity is limited to an area of the brain that is vital to speech, the surgery will not be undertaken. Surgery is especially effective when the medial temporal lobe on one side or a structural defect (detectable with magnetic resonance imaging) can be identified as the source of seizures. For many people with intractable seizures, surgery is a reasonable option when medications have had little or no impact on the epilepsy.

Some neurosurgeons have attempted to manage seizures arising from several regions of the brain by cutting the corpus callosum—the bundle of nerve fibers that make up the principal connection between the two sides of the brain. Cutting the corpus callosum prevents disruptive signals that originate on one side of the brain from spreading to the other side. This type of surgery is effective for a few highly selected people, mostly ones who suffer from epileptic drop attacks. Whether it could be beneficial for a particular person with intractable seizures is a decision that must involve both the neurosurgeon who will do the procedure and a neurologist who is thoroughly familiar with the patient's disorder.

Vagus Nerve Stimulation

In this procedure, a major nerve that courses down the neck into the chest—the vagus nerve—is connected to a pacemaker-like device that is implanted under the skin. This pacemaker serves as an electrical stimulator; shocks transmitted up this nerve to the brain apparently interfere with seizures. The device is usually programmed to stimulate for 30 seconds and then turn off for 5 minutes, 24 hours a day. The person may also activate the stimulator using a magnet that is placed over the skin where the stimulator is implanted.

This approach works best for people who have partial seizures with auras that give them an opportunity to activate the device. The long-term value of vagus nerve stimulation remains to be established, but it appears to be useful in people with partial and perhaps generalized seizures for whom medications have not worked. Attempts to suppress seizures with direct electrical stimulation of nerve tissues have not been of clear benefit, though experience with this technique is limited.

Informed Consent for Brain Surgery

Surgery on the brain to stop seizures, like any other form of neurosurgery, involves substantial risks and is generally appropriate only when the person (or guardian) can fully understand the risks and when all other reasonable options have been exhausted. Infections, bleeding, further brain damage, and even death from anesthesia are all possible in the most competent hands. Some families, exhausted and frustrated after years of recurrent seizures, will exert subtle or not-so-subtle pressure on the person with seizures to submit to surgery. Conversely, an overprotective family occasionally tries to block the patient's decision to have surgery.

Because no neurologist or neurosurgeon can guarantee that the surgery will control seizures and will not produce new problems, the decision to take these risks must be strictly the patient's. Similarly, patients for whom surgery is appropriate must be given access to this treatment if they want it and if they are competent to weigh the potential costs and benefits.

The need for thoroughly informed consent presents obvious problems in dealing with a child who might profit from seizure surgery. A 9-year-old who has had poorly controlled seizures for five years is not competent to decide the appropriateness of neurosurgery. Intellectual development is often significantly impaired by recurrent seizures, and the outlook for improvement is bleak as long as the seizures remain poorly controlled.

The child's parents must make an exceedingly difficult decision. If they agree to the surgery, they may feel responsible for an unsatisfactory result; but if they reject the procedure, they may suffer considerable guilt as they watch the child continue to have frequent seizures and to fall hopelessly behind her peer group. If there are other children in the family, they may be neglected as the parents agonize over whether to subject the epileptic child to surgery. If one parent is less convinced than the other that surgery is essential, the more agreeable parent may be blamed if the surgery produces less than excellent results. Confounding every decision to perform surgery is the possibility, however remote, that a newly introduced medication will eliminate the seizures without damaging or removing brain tissue.

In any decision involving neurosurgery on a child, it is essential that the entire family have an opportunity to air questions, fears, and misconceptions. This is not an emergency procedure, and so there is time to allow the parents and other family members to reach a consensus. The fact is that brain surgery in a child with poorly controlled seizures is sometimes very effective, and neurologic deficits appearing after the surgery are often transient. A physician with no vested interest in the procedure—that is, one who will not be involved in the surgery and has no affiliation with the center performing the surgery—should discuss the advisability of the procedure with the family.

If surgery is chosen, the purpose and character of the surgery should not be concealed from the epileptic child. Efforts to protect the child by keeping her in the dark can lead her to develop terrifying fantasies to explain the ordeal.

Diets, Vitamins, and Homeopathic Cures

Everyone faced with a lifelong burden of medication or uncertain seizure control hopes for a simple cure. This accounts for the enduring appeal of special diets, vitamin regimens, and other remedies ranging from religious ceremonies to exercise classes. An eyewitness account of a remarkable cure or a dramatic improvement in seizure control is more convincing than bland statistics showing that the effect of the megavitamins, holy water, biofeedback, or self-hypnosis does not exceed what would have been expected on the basis of chance alone. The inexplicable treatment has the allure of magic. After dealing with negative or blasé doctors, people find it a relief to hear from proselytizing faddists that little more than an act of faith will cure them.

Logic does not usually discourage a person with epilepsy from pursuing these unorthodox treatments. The best that anyone can hope for is that the person will not discontinue an effective treatment in a misguided effort to pursue a simpler remedy.

One diet that does help with seizure control has been recognized for decades. This is the ketogenic diet, which is high in fats and low in carbohydrates and protein. Raising the level of ketones in the blood by eating a diet consisting mostly of vegetable oils and cream will reduce the seizure threshold in many people, but the foods allowed are difficult to tolerate even for a few days, and to be effective the diet must be followed for longer periods.

The ketogenic diet is used as a supplement to antiepileptic medication in children with minor motor seizures when drugs have failed to suppress seizures. It is a dietary approach with documented merit, but the character of the diet makes it unacceptable except for the most desperate people. Experience with this treatment strategy in adults is extremely limited, and the risks are poorly understood.

Group Therapy

Whether people with epilepsy choose medication, surgery, or dietary fads to control their seizures, they and their families usually profit from the opportunity to meet with similarly affected people. Such interactions eliminate the feeling of isolation that often burdens people who have a seizure disorder. In group meetings, the deception and fear of discovery that permeate the life of a person with marginally controlled epilepsy can be discarded. Discussing the problems associated with work, family, seizure control, and sexual dysfunction can be very helpful, because people with similar types of epilepsy often have remarkably similar problems.

Self-deprecation is common when a person with epilepsy first enters group discussions, but after a few meetings this attitude abates. People feel less impaired when they see what other people with similar problems have done. Alliances develop quickly, and from them strategies for dealing with epilepsy are learned.

The animosity that often characterizes the interactions between people with epilepsy and their unaffected peers also abates under the influence of group therapy. People with almost any chronic disability tend to harbor some resentment, jealousy, and self-pity, but these feelings decrease substantially when affected individuals are able to get together regularly to talk about their mutual problems.

When family members are involved in the group, the strains that have developed within the family tend to lessen. In one typical family group that met on a regular basis for several months, the most common issues raised included adjusting to the illness, relieving tension in the family, planning the future, balancing dangers faced willingly by the person with the desire to feel useful, financial worries, divorce, suicide, changes in social life, living in the present, medication compliance, explaining the illness to other people, dealing with doctors, alternatives to work, and problems with the immediate and extended family.

All of these issues require attention, and solutions to them will not be found in a doctor's office. Finding alternatives to a lifestyle that has had to be abandoned because of a seizure disorder is not the function of a physician; the alternatives must come from people who have the problem. Similarly, figuring out ways to adjust family life to the demands of epilepsy cannot be accomplished in an office visit. Families need to meet one another and have opportunities to explore coping strategies in a low-stress setting. Involving medical personnel in the meeting sometimes helps to counteract the erroneous information brought by participating families, and involving a family therapist may direct the group to real insights.

Most families can survive the disruptiveness of epilepsy in one of its members, but no family struggling under this burden should be expected to function productively alone.

Chapter Twelve

What To Do When a Seizure Occurs

When a seizure occurs, family members are often obliged to cope with it. If an isolated seizure occurs in a person who has a well-established seizure disorder, there is usually no need to get emergency medical attention. But if the episode is a change in the person's usual level of seizure control, the physician should be notified.

There is little that anyone—physician, family member, or Good Samaritan—can do during the seizure to stop it; this is important to remember when people witnessing the seizure run about frantically and insist that something must be done. The principal objective is to keep the person having the seizure from suffering any injury (see Table 29). If the seizure is a generalized absence (petit mal) episode, the risk of self-injury is negligible. If the seizure is a generalized tonic-clonic (grand mal) seizure or progresses to a generalized convulsion, the risk of injury is much more substantial. People with focal motor or focal sensory seizures may need no assistance during the episode. People with confusion during the ictal phase, but no

TABLE 29
How to Help during a Grand Mal Seizure

Do:	Do not:
Help him lie down on his side	Struggle to open his jaws
Put padding around his head	Place a finger in his mouth
Move nearby objects	Force anything between his teeth
Get him to an emergency room if status epilepticus occurs	Give him something to drink while he is still confused

motor problems such as falling to the ground or thrashing limbs, may need little more than careful observation and occasional direction to avoid mishaps.

Avoiding Restraints

Trying to restrain convulsive movements of the limbs or trunk can injure both the person having the seizure and the person restraining him; it is unnecessary and unwise. Rather than holding the victim's arms and legs, bystanders should try to clear objects out of his way. A person with convulsive seizures who realizes that a seizure is about to occur should be helped into a position that will minimize the danger of injury. The ideal position is lying on the side in the middle of a padded floor without furniture or other objects nearby to fall against or kick. There is little point in having the person lie on a narrow sofa or sit in a padded chair, since he is likely to fall off.

With seizures that involve little thrashing about and much strenuous posturing, pillows placed under or around the victim may reduce bruising. If the person is already unconscious and lying on his back when he is found, it is often a good idea to roll him onto his side to keep him from choking. When changing the person's position, one should push or pull on the trunk, not the limbs, because shoulder dislocations sometimes occur during generalized convulsions.

Limited Use of Tongue Protection

Never force a spoon, stick, or other object into the mouth of a person who is having a seizure. If the jaws are firmly closed, trying to pry them apart with a stiff object may cause more damage than the convulsion itself. Teeth may be dislodged and end up in the lungs, and the tongue or gums may be lacerated. If there is warning that a generalized convulsion is going to occur, a thin but strong and well-padded object, such as a wooden tongue depressor wrapped with gauze, can be placed between the jaws to keep them from closing completely. This may protect the tongue and gums from being bitten. Dentures or other removable dental work should be removed if there is time at the beginning of a seizure.

Avoiding Assisted Breathing

During generalized convulsions breathing may stop for several seconds or appear very labored, and the person may turn slightly blue. These changes make witnesses worry that the seizure victim will suffocate. Observers should not attempt to clear the victim's airway. In a minute or two, as the ictus passes, the victim will develop a more normal skin color and breathing pattern. If breathing remains disturbed and the mouth can be opened, obstruction of the airway should be cautiously but rapidly investigated by gently pulling the tongue forward and tilting the head backward. The seizure victim cannot actually "swallow" his tongue, but it may partially obstruct the airway. If the impaired consciousness is from a seizure, resuscitation should not be necessary.

Avoiding Aspiration

Trying to get the seizure victim to drink immediately after the convulsion is dangerous. The liquid may be inhaled into the lungs, and the cough reflex that would normally limit the damage that such aspirated fluid could cause in the lungs is likely to be defective during the early postictal period. There is no beverage, alcoholic or otherwise, that will speed the victim's recovery from the confusion that follows a seizure.

Avoiding Premature Activity

Rushing the seizure victim into walking or sitting before the postictal confusion has cleared is also risky. Although seeing the person upright may be reassuring to bystanders, it increases the possibility of a fall. The victim will get up without encouragement when the confusion has passed. If an injury, such as a twisted ankle or a pulled back muscle, has occurred during the seizure, the person can avoid making it worse much more effectively when he is fully alert than when he is confused.

Recognizing Status Epilepticus

When seizures occur one after another with no return to normal consciousness in between, the person is said to be in status epilepticus. This is a potentially lethal situation if competent medical treatment is not quickly obtained. In the hands of an experienced neurologist or other physician familiar with its management, status epilepticus is usually completely reversible.

Two or three seizures in one day do not constitute status epilepticus, but four or five seizures in one hour are highly suggestive of the problem. Also, since grand mal seizures rarely last more than two minutes, status epilepticus should be suspected whenever a seizure lasts longer than five minutes. Anyone having frequent or prolonged seizures should be brought to a facility equipped to manage status epilepticus. In most cases, this means a hospital emergency room.

Treatment Changes

Changes in medication on the day that a seizure occurs should always be decided by the patient's physician. Family members often give the person additional medication immediately after a seizure. The rate at which most antiepileptic drugs are absorbed into the bloodstream is too slow to make this a useful strategy in most cases. Notable exceptions include carbamazepine, primidone, and valproate, but the dosages of these medications may already be at maximum beneficial levels when seizures recur, and increasing the number of pills taken may be useless.

Because seizures may occur at inopportune times and physicians cannot always be contacted when urgent questions arise, the people who are likely to be present when the person has a seizure should have a clearly defined plan. What should be done about medication on the day of the seizure, what signs justify a trip to the emergency room, and what questions should be asked after the seizure to help define its cause should all be settled before the seizure occurs, in consultation with the physician.

Suggested Reading and References

General Information

Commission on Classification and Terminology of the International League Against Epilepsy. "Proposal for the classification of epilepsy and epileptic syndromes." *Epilepsia* 30 (1989):389–399.

Dreifuss, Fritz E. "Seizure disorders." In *Current Practice of Medicine*, ed. Roger C. Bone: vol. 3, ed. William C. Koller. New York: Churchill Livingstone, 1996.

Engel, Jerome, Jr. *Seizures and Epilepsy.* Philadelphia: Davis, 1989.

Lechtenberg, Richard. *Seizure Recognition and Treatment.* New York: Churchill Livingstone, 1990.

Lechtenberg, Richard, and Henry S. Schutta, eds. *Neurology Practice Guidelines.* New York: Marcel Dekker, 1998.

Treatment of Epilepsy

Ballaban-Gil, K., C. Callahan, C. O'Dell, M. Pappo, et al. "Complications of the ketogenic diet." *Epilepsia* 39 (1998):744–748.

Brodie, M. J., and M. A. Dichter. "Drug therapy: antiepileptic drugs." *New England Journal of Medicine* 334 (1996):168–175.

Brodie, M. J., and John M. Pellock. "Taming the brain storms: felbamate updated." *Lancet* 346 (1996):918–919.

Duchowny, M., P. Jayakar, T. Resnick, A. S. Harvey, et al. "Epilepsy surgery in the first three years of life." *Epilepsia* 39 (1989):737–743.

"Felbamate." *Medical Letter for Drugs and Therapeutics* 35 (1993):107–109.

Fernandez, R. J., and M. A. Samuels. "Epilepsy," in *Manual of Neurologic Therapeutics*, 5th ed., ed. M. A. Samuels. Boston: Little, Brown, 1994.

"Gabapentin—a new anticonvulsant." *Medical Letter for Drugs and Therapeutics* 36 (1994):39–40.

Handforth A., C. M. DeGiorgio, S. C. Schachter, B. M. Uthman, et al. "Vagus nerve stimulation therapy for partial-onset seizures: a randomized active-control trial." *Neurology* 51 (1998):48–55.

Kraemer, D. L., M. L. Griebel, N. Lee, A. H. Friedman, and R. A. Radtke. "Surgical outcome in patients with epilepsy with occult vascular malformations treated with lesionectomy." *Epilepsia* 39 (1998):600–607.

Montouris, G. D. "Practical insights and clinical experience with combinations of the new antiepileptic drugs." *Neurology* 45, suppl. 2 (1995):S25–S28.

Pellock, John M. "Antiepileptic drug therapy in the United States: a review of clinical studies and unmet needs." *Neurology* 45, suppl. 2 (1995):S17–S24.

Read, C. L., L. J. Stephen, I. H. Stolareck, et al. "Cognitive effects of anticonvulsant monotherapy in elderly patients: a placebo-controlled study." *Seizure* 7 (1998):159–162.

Sandok, E. K., and G. D. Cascino. "Surgical treatment for perirolandic lesional epilepsy." *Epilepsia* 39, suppl. 4 (1998):S42–S48.

Wilder, B. J. "The treatment of epilepsy: an overview of clinical practices." *Neurology* 45, suppl. 2 (1995):S7–S11.

Wyllie, E., ed. *The Treatment of Epilepsy: Principles and Practice.* Philadelphia: Lea and Febiger, 1993.

The Adult with Epilepsy

Lechtenberg, R., and Dana Ohl. *Sexual Dysfunction*. Philadelphia: Lea and Febiger, 1994.

Meade, T. W. "Risk of recurrent seizures." *New England Journal of Medicine* 339 (1998):128–129.

Sillanpaa, M., M. Jalava, O. Kaleva, and S. Shinnar. "Long-term prognosis of seizures with onset in childhood." *New England Journal of Medicine* 338 (1998):1715–1722.

Verity, C. M., et al. "Long-term intellectual and behavioral outcomes of children with febrile convulsions." *New England Journal of Medicine* 338 (1998):1723–1728.

Willmore, L. J. "Antiepileptic drug therapy in the elderly." *Pharmacology and Therapeutics* 78 (1998):9–16.

Yagi, K. "Epilepsy: comprehensive care, quality of life, and factors preventing people with epilepsy from being employed." *Clinical Therapeutics* 20 (1998):A19–A29.

Childbearing and Inheritance

Delgado-Escueta, A. V., and D. Janz. "Consensus guidelines: preconception counseling, management, and care of the pregnant woman with epilepsy." *Neurology* 42, suppl. 5 (1992):149–160.

Dichter, M. A., and J. R. Buchhalter. "The genetic epilepsies." In *The Molecular and Genetic Basis of Neurological Disease*, ed. R. Rosenberg, S. Prusiner, S. DiMaura, R. Barchi, and L. Kunkel. Boston: Butterworth-Heinemann, 1993.

Duncan, S., J. Blacklaw, G. H. Beastall, and M. J. Brodie. "Sexual function in women with epilepsy." *Epilepsia* 38 (1998):1074–1081.

Kaneko, S. "Pregnancy and quality of life in women with epilepsy." *Clinical Therapeutics* 20, suppl. A (1998):A30–A47.

Morrell, M. J. "Issues for women with epilepsy." *Western Journal of Medicine* 168 (1998):266–267.

Pintz, C. "Prescribing medication in pregnancy." *Lippincott's Primary Care Practice* 2 (1998):230–240.

Swartjes, J. M., and H. P. Geijn. "Pregnancy and epilepsy." *European Journal of Obstetrics & Gynecology and Reproductive Biology* 79 (1998):3–11.

Yerby, M. S. "Teratogenic effects of antiepileptic drugs: what do we advise patients?" *Epilepsia* 38 (1997):957–958.

Children with Epilepsy

Caviedes, B. E., and J. L. Herranz. "Seizure recurrence and risk factors after withdrawal of chronic antiepileptic therapy in children." *Seizure* 7 (1998):107–114.

Dreifuss, Fritz E. "Prognosis of childhood seizure disorders: present and future." *Epilepsia* 34 (1994):S30–S34.

Ettinger, A. B., D. M. Weisbrot, E. E. Nolan, K. D. Gadow, et al. "Symptoms of depression and anxiety in pediatric epilepsy patients." *Epilepsia* 39 (1998):595–599.

Kokkonen, E. R., J. Kokkonen, and A. L. Saukkonen. "Do neurological disorders in childhood pose a risk for mental health in young adulthood?" *Developmental Medicine and Child Neurology* 40 (1998):364–368.

Mukahira, K., H. Oguni, Y. Awaya, et al. "Study of surgical treatment of intractable childhood epilepsy." *Brain Development* 20 (1998):154–164.

Roger, J., M. Bureau, C. Dravet, et al. *Epileptic Syndromes in Infancy, Childhood, and Adolescence.* London: John Libbey, 1992.

Vining, E. P. "Gaining a perspective on childhood seizures." *New England Journal of Medicine* 338 (1998):1916–1918.

Wirrell, E. C. "Benign epilepsy of childhood with centrotemporal spikes." *Epilepsia* 39, suppl. 4 (1989):S32–S41.

Psychologic Features

Bredkjaer, S. R., P. B. Mortensen, and J. Parnas. "Epilepsy and non-organic non-affective psychosis: national epidemiologic study." *British Journal of Psychiatry* 172 (1998):235–238.

Carlton-Ford, S., R. Miller, N. Nealeigh, and N. Sanchez. "The effects of perceived stigma and psychological over-control on the behavioural problems of children with epilepsy." *Seizure* 6 (1997):383–391.

Devinsky, O. "Nonepileptic psychogenic seizures: quagmires of pathophysiology, diagnosis, and treatment." *Epilepsia* 39 (1998):458–462.

Henry, T., and I. Drury. "Ictal behaviors during nonepileptic seizures differ in patients with temporal lobe interictal epileptiform
EEG activity and patients without interictal epileptiform abnormalities." *Epilepsia* 39 (1998):175–182.

Newsom-Davis, I., L. H. Goldstein, and D. Fitzpatrick. "Fear of seizures: an investigation and treatment." *Seizures* 7 (1998):101–
106.

Mortality

George, J. R., and G. G. Davis. "Comparison of anti-epileptic drug
levels in different cases of sudden death." *Journal of Forensic
Science* 43 (1998):598–603.

Natelson, B. H., R. V. Suarez, C. F. Terrence, and R. Turizo. "Patients with epilepsy who die suddenly have cardiac disease." *Ar-
chives of Neurology* 55 (1998):857–860.

Nilsson, L., T. Tomson, B. Y. Farahmand, V. Diwan, and P. G.
Persson. "Cause-specific mortality in epilepsy: a cohort study of
more than 9,000 patients once hospitalized for epilepsy."
Epilepsia 38 (1997):1062–1068.

Index

Figures and tables are referred to with f and t, respectively.